PERSONALIZED

PARKINSON'S

Maximize Your Health by

Individualizing Your Care

Dr. Ben Weinstock

Foreword by Dr. Rudy Capildeo

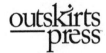
outskirts
press

Medical Information Disclaimer

The information and reference materials contained here are intended solely for the general information of the reader. It is not to be used for treatment purposes, but rather for discussion with the patient's own physician. The information presented here is not intended to diagnose health problems or to take the place of professional medical care. The information contained herein is neither intended to dictate what constitutes reasonable, appropriate or best care for any given health issue, nor is it intended to be used as a substitute for the independent judgment of a physician for any given health issue. All content is for general information purposes only. If you have persistent health problems or if you have further questions, please consult your health care provider. Reference to any products, services, hypertext link to the third parties or other information by trade name, trademark, supplier or otherwise does not constitute or imply its endorsement, sponsorship or recommendation by the author or owner of the copyright. They are for convenience only. This book does not constitute an attempt to practice medicine. The use of this book and any related materials does not establish a doctor-patient relationship. Individuals should consult a qualified health care provider for medical advice and answers to personal health questions. The primary responsibility of your disease management plan is with your treating physicians and you should only follow your treating physician's advice. DO NOT change/modify your disease management plan on your own without consulting your treating physicians. While the author has attempted to be as accurate as possible, his work should not be relied upon as being comprehensive or error-free.

Me, we.

— Muhammad Ali

Dedication

This book is dedicated to the millions of people around the world diagnosed with Parkinson's Disease, and to their caregivers.

I hope the information in this book can help to relieve some of their trials and tribulations.

Foreword

As a medical student at St. George's Hospital, Hyde Park Corner, London in the mid-1960's Parkinson's Disease (PD) was a medical oddity. Historically a fascinating story but with no effective treatment, PD occupied little space in the neurological curriculum. "What are the causes of Parkinson's?" We would answer "drug-induced" and "idiopathic;" in other words, "we did not know." "What are the cardinal features?" The immediate reply might be "tremor, rigidity, bradykinesia."

Clearly, we had not read James Parkinson's "Essay on the Shaking Palsy" which he had published himself in 1817. If we had then we would have known his wonderful description of the gait disorder which I bring up to date as follows: the loss of the heel-strike (the foot-brake), walking on the fore-part of the foot, (the accelerator), the tendency to lean and run forward (festinant gait), even to fall if not caught. To this we can add the characteristic posture with forward stoop, knees slightly bent and already on the toes, loss of arm swing, difficulty turning and difficulties in maintaining balance. Perhaps the most important facet, however, is the initial delay before movement is initiated, the most frustrating pause for the PD person, the caregiver or the medical attendant.

James Parkinson was describing a MOVEMENT DISORDER. He thought all patients had a tremor (but only about 50% of patients have it) hence "Shaking" and the slowness and stiffness, and "Palsy" (a type of paralysis). His little book is remarkable. James was a General Practitioner in Shoreditch, East London. He described 3 patients he saw in his clinic at 1 Hoxton Square and 3 people he recognised in the street with the same condition. Importantly, he also said that the condition usually began asymmetrically (not yet explained) and that the intellect and "senses" were not involved. This excludes those other conditions that have some parkinsonian features, cognitive disturbances and dementia.

It was very fortunate that the famous physician Dr Jean-Martin Charcot found a copy of the book and immediately recognised the condition in his native Paris, Amsterdam, London and "everywhere I went." Known as the founder of the Clinical Speciality of Neurology, it was Charcot who recommended that this condition should be called "Parkinson's Disease."

Parkinson's is common. More than 1 person in 70 has this over the age of 70 years. The usual patient in the clinic has a "Dopamine Depletion Disorder" (my term) which can be quickly helped with low-dose L-Dopa medication (Sinemet, introduced in 1973 and Madopar in 1974). Since the average patient has had their condition undiagnosed for up to 5 years, there is an awful lot to catch up on and improve. The new medication is to supplement and not suppress the patient's own, albeit reduced, endogenous production of dopamine.

At the new Charing Cross Hospital, Fulham, London, I was appointed the first Registrar in Neurology. It was 1st May 1973. I remember the day a representative from Merck Sharp and Dohme Pharmaceuticals walked in and said "I've got a special drug for you!" With the advent of Sinemet we opened the first Parkinson's Disease Clinic in West London. All the focus was on medication, medication and medication. Then studies were published about the use of exercise in Parkinson's. These studies taught me that the secret to long-term wellness was a personalised approach towards the care of any individual with Parkinson's, the ongoing interaction between a Parkinson's patient with a positive attitude, a caregiver who encourages the patient everyday and the help of a dedicated healthcare professional. This can be difficult to achieve since every patient is an individual with individual needs. Caregivers have to respond to daily needs of their loved ones and to respond quickly when reaching out to appropriate Healthcare Professionals. In so doing, the care of the patient becomes efficient and personalised.

I know that the care of a person with Parkinson's can be extremely difficult due to a multitude of problems that may arise (more complicated than simply a movement disorder), with the vast amount of media interest, different treatment options and greater public awareness. For this reason, *Personalized Parkinson's: Maximize Your Health by Individualizing Your Care*, is invaluable. Each chapter provides cutting-edge research not only for optimizing care, but also for spotting issues before they become more serious. Each topic – from diet to exercise to sleep, and many others – is geared towards maintaining and improving one's quality of life with Parkinson's Disease. You or your caregiver can use this book to formulate questions for the members of your healthcare team. Consider it to be your guidebook for personalized care.

Dr. Rudy Capildeo, FRCP,
Consultant Neurologist
United Kingdom

About Dr. Ben Weinstock

Dr. Ben Weinstock, PT, DPT, C-LIFE is a Doctor of Physical Therapy with more than 30 years of experience. He specializes in treating patients with neurodegenerative diseases and complex medical conditions. After finishing his Doctorate in Physical Therapy, he completed a Certification in Health Focused Lifestyle Intervention. He is a member of several scientific organizations including the International Parkinson and Movement Disorder Society. Dr. Weinstock is the developer and teacher of EPIC-PD (Exercise Prescription, Individualized Care) ™, a personalized exercise and lifestyle approach based on a patient's neurovascular responses to exercise. He has presented his work at international meetings and was named as a Committee Member of the International Conference on Parkinson's Disease and Movement Disorders. In 2015 he published *Preventing Parkinson's: How to Cut Your Risk by Strengthening Your Multiple Shields*, the first and only book about the prevention of the disease.

About Dr. Rudy Capildeo

Dr. Rudy Capildeo has been a Consultant Neurologist in the United Kingdom for over 50 years. He has extensive experience treating Parkinson's Disease and other neurological conditions; as well as teaching, writing, and participating in clinical research and drug development. He is recognized internationally as an expert clinician.

Table of Contents

1

You and the Scope of Parkinson's Disease

If you are reading this book, the chances are that you have been diagnosed with Parkinson's Disease (PD).

You have probably thought, "What can I do to stay as healthy as possible? How can I still lead a good life?"

This book was written for you.

Whenever possible, I have provided information to help you make sure that your healthcare is individualized as much as possible. "Personalized medicine" usually refers to treatments based on the integration of genetics, environmental, lifestyle, and clinical information. It is also referred to as "precision medicine."[1]

To use the analogy of getting eyeglasses: when you go to an eye care professional, he or she does not simply reach into a drawer and hand you a pair of eyeglasses and state, "Take these glasses…this prescription works for some of my patients."

A generic pair of eyeglasses *might* help you, but most likely the result would be less than satisfactory. And the generic eyeglasses might even make your vision worse. What would help you the most would be a true eyeglass <u>prescription</u>.

In many ways, lifestyle interventions for PD are generic and not bad overall, but they are not specific enough for an individual with PD.

For example, group exercise classes for PD rarely take each individual's exercise tolerance (or intolerance) into account. Very often, the standard recommendations of moderate to intensive exercise, up to one hour a day, may be good for the *prevention* of PD, but once someone develops the condition, what is good for prevention is not the same as for *treating* the condition. The reason: the body undergoes changes in a disease state. Moreover, each person has their own unique presentation of PD. As we will discuss in the chapter about exercise, there are many PD-related factors that may influence the safety of exercise, such as changes in blood pressure, heart rate, and body temperature.

The same can be discussed about diet. One person with PD may be able to tolerate certain foods, but once the disease state sets in, new problems may arise. These can include difficulty chewing, delayed swallowing, slow emptying of the stomach, and constipation. Obviously, a person with such problems need the intervention of specialists, not a simple diet plan downloaded from a website.

Estimates vary as to how many people in the United States have PD (and related disorders)—somewhere between one to one and a half million. Worldwide, there are between seven to ten million people with PD.[2] The disease strikes men more than women. This is probably due not only to the hormonal differences between the sexes, but also because of higher industrial exposures for men as compared to women.[3]

Approximately 60,000 people are diagnosed with PD each year in America.[4] Although the majority of these cases are "typical PD," there are also "atypical" types. Moreover, as knowledge about brain diseases continues to advance, there is a greater appreciation that there are many sub-types of PD and PD-related conditions.[5]

There is also a growing awareness of the many conditions that mimic PD. Some of these mimics include DIP

(Drug Induced Parkinson's); PD caused by small strokes (Vascular Parkinson's); a variety of diseases that cause tremors; as well as other neurological conditions. In a recent poll conducted by Parkinsons UK of over 2,000 people, more than a quarter of them reported that they were initially misdiagnosed. The dangers of being misdiagnosed: they were treated with Parkinson's medications that were not needed; some received medications and neurosurgery.[6] Although this misdiagnosis rate seems unusually high, other studies have shown that the initial misdiagnosis rate can be as high as 75%.[7]

Clearly, PD is not easy to diagnose. Movement disorder specialists probably have the highest accuracy in making the diagnosis. If they have doubts, they may consider a specialized brain study. One such test is a type of brain imaging technique called DaTscan. The results of a DaTscan can raise the correct diagnosis rate, and lower the misdiagnosis rate.[8] Other types of tests are also under review, and show great promise in ensuring that the diagnosis of PD is even more accurate: biopsies of skin, colon, or submandibular gland.[9]

The healthcare costs of PD are staggering: the disease costs 25 billion dollars a year in America, including medications, treatments, disability payments, and lost wages.[10] It has been estimated that with the aging of the population, the numbers are expected to double by the year 2030.[11] However, according to Dr. Caroline Tanner (one of the world's leading PD experts), it may actually be worse: the projected doubling of the cases of PD worldwide is based solely on aging.[12]

Therefore, what we have is a complex, multi-faceted disease which is expected to become much more prevalent in coming years. Moreover, there is a lack of resources that discuss how to truly individualize care for people diagnosed with PD.

THE MULTIPLE HIT THEORY OF PD

The number one risk factor for developing PD is aging.[13] If someone develops PD before the age of 50, it is considered "Young-Onset Parkinson's Disease." Cases of Young Onset Parkinson's Disease represent between 3% - 6% of all cases of PD.[14]

The overwhelming majority of PD cases are considered "sporadic" or "typical" and are diagnosed over the age of 50. From that point forward, the risk of developing PD continues to increases with age.[15] PD affects about 1-2%

of people aged 65 and older, but this goes up to more than 4% of people who are 85 and older.[16]

One of the neurotransmitters (chemical messengers) lost in PD is dopamine. Dopamine has a multitude of functions in the brain. Not only does it ensure smooth movements, but it is also a key player in learning, motivation, and reward-seeking behaviors.[17]

It is estimated that we lose at least 5% of our dopamine levels with each decade over the age of 40.[18] The longer we live, the less dopamine we have. About 50% of people aged 85 and older have *Parkinsonism* – a condition that can be characterized by mild tremor, trouble walking, poor balance, and slowness of movement. But they do not necessarily have PD. Their problems are probably due to lower levels of other neurotransmitters besides dopamine.[19]

We cannot blame all cases of PD simply on aging. Not every elderly person develops PD. But it appears that aging, combined with certain genetic vulnerabilities and environmental exposures, leads to PD in susceptible individuals.[20] The combination of unhealthy vulnerabilities and exposures is referred to as *multiple hits*. These multiple hits may be: poor diet; poor sleep; head trauma;

lack of exercise; stress; exposure to toxins; and other un-healthy factors.

Combat veterans illustrate the impact of multiple hits. They have more than twice the risk of developing PD as compared to non-combat veterans and civilians.[21] It was found that soldiers who survived prisoner of war camps during World War Two developed PD and other neuro-logical conditions 30-35 years later at a rate much higher than in the normal population.[22] This may be due to the multiple hits that soldiers may suffer, such as severe men-tal stress, head injuries, poor nutrition, infections,[23] and possible chemical exposures.[24] Unfortunately, the effects continue for many veterans after they are discharged. The combination of post-traumatic stress disorder (PTSD), sleep disorders,[25] and overall poor health[26] adds up to higher risks of diseases for combat veterans.

ALPHA-SYNUCLEIN: THE NORMAL PROTEIN THAT BECOMES ABNORMAL

The culprit that appears to be the cause of PD is the buildup of a protein within brain cells. This protein, al-pha-synuclein, is naturally occurring. In fact, it is an im-portant part of normal nerve function, probably in the

release and maintenance of *vesicles* (microscopic pack-
ages) of neurotransmitters.[27]

Unfortunately, abnormalities of alpha-synuclein have
the potential to cause major problems. There may be a
genetic explanation (such as an inherited excess of the
protein), or a mixture of genes and environment (triggering misshapen, clumped-together versions of the protein). If alpha-synuclein builds up, it can disrupt normal
cell activity in many ways. There is evidence that it
causes, directly or indirectly: defects in dopamine vesicles;[28] interference with the energy-producing machinery of the cell; inhibition of the recycling processes of the
cell; blockage of the transmission of chemical messengers; generation of high levels of free radicals;[29] interference with other proteins; and disturbance of the
architecture of cells.[30] Abnormal alpha-synuclein multi-
plies toxic reactions within cells by a factor of *more than
1,000.*[31] The body responds to damage by attempting to
regenerate nerve pathways; however, alpha-synuclein inhibits this process.[32] Moreover, extremely high levels of
alpha-synuclein appear to lower the threshold for responses to environmental stressors. For example, manganese (which is needed by the body in trace amounts) is
considered to be a toxin when exposures are long-term,

and/or excessive. But high levels of alpha-synuclein make even lower levels of manganese toxic.[33]

DR. BRAAK'S THEORY OF PD

A theory of how PD begins, and spreads, was proposed by the neuroanatomist Dr. Heiko Braak.[34] He and his team discovered that the disease is initiated in various regions of the brain (via the nasal passages) as well as in the gut.[35] Alpha-synuclein formation proceeds in stages, where it "infects" other cells. This domino-like effect proceeds from the gut to the brain along the longest nerve in the body, the vagus nerve.[36] Although Dr. Braak's proposed staging of the disease has been criticized,[37] it is still a valid guideline for understanding the spread of PD in most patients.

The motor and non-motor problems of PD; the timeline of Parkinson's Disease

You may be familiar with the fable of the king who asked a group of blind men to examine an elephant. One blind man touched the elephant's tail, and reported that the elephant was like a rope. Another blind man touched the elephant's tusk, and stated that the animal was like a curved pipe. The blind man who touched one of the elephant's ears disagreed with the others, saying that the elephant was like a large fan. And the blind man who touched the elephant's leg proclaimed that the others were all wrong—the elephant was like a tree trunk. Of course, the king informed them that they were all correct—but only by combining their individual observations. This is not unlike the multiple aspects of PD. There is a wide variety in how PD will present itself. Although the basic core of the disease is similar, the overall presentation among people suffering from PD can be vastly different. Neurologists have proposed that because there is no single version of "Parkinson's Disease" the condition should be called *Parkinson Diseases* [38] or *Parkinson's Disease Cluster.*[39]

Because there is no single version of PD, care must be tailored for each unique case of PD.

People with PD develop problems, generally classified into motor (movement-related) signs, and non-motor signs:

Motor signs: tremor, rigidity, slowness of movement, balance problems, gait dysfunction, freezing of gait, postural problems (forward or sideways trunk lean), difficulty swallowing, difficulty speaking, and a mask-like face.

Non-motor signs: gastrointestinal (such as constipation), genitourinary (bladder problems, sexual difficulties), sleep disorders, cardiovascular (including low blood pressure, irregular heartbeats, poor exercise response), thermoregulatory (increased or decreased sweating), neuropsychiatric (such as depression, apathy, cognitive impairment, dementia, hallucinations), sensory changes (including pain, loss of smell, numbness, visual disturbances), fatigue, weight changes.

Not everyone develops all of the above listed problems. Some people have relatively mild symptoms; others have to face more challenges.

When is someone diagnosed with PD? It is usually once the *motor* signs begin to appear. It is estimated that the motor signs are caused by a loss of dopamine-producing cells of at least 50%.[40] It may start with a tremor. Or maybe the first sign is difficulty walking. Or it could be repeated falls. Eventually the person is seen by a primary care physician. With further questioning, "the big picture" begins to emerge. What problems has the patient been dealing with over the past few years, or decades? Constipation? Depression? Sleep problems? Fatigue?

These (and other) non-motor problems are part of what is called the pre-PD, or *preclinical* phase. This means that the disease was there, slowly damaging various bodily functions, before the patient showed the typical motor signs of PD.

The non-motor problems begin in regions of the brain that produce various neurotransmitters, such as norepinephrine, serotonin, GABA, and acetylcholine. When the disease spreads to the region of the brain that produces dopamine, the motor problems begin. This explains the progression, over time, of preclinical non-motor problems to motor problems.[41]

Back to our patient: the primary care physician (who probably has a strong suspicion that it is PD) will refer the patient to a neurologist, who rules out any conditions that may mimic PD. If the final diagnosis is indeed PD, the patient will be prescribed anti-PD medications. As the disease progresses, other treatments (such as Deep Brain Stimulation) may be considered.

NEUROPROTECTION

Current interventions for PD can be called *neuroprotective*: treatments that aim to protect the nervous system against further harm. You can try to maximize your body's defenses. You can try to minimize the problems associated with PD.

Just as multiple hits conspire together to trigger PD, fortifying our multiple lines of defense may be able to lower the risk of developing PD-related dysfunctions. The popularity of this concept has been growing in recent years, especially among drug researchers. Instead of looking for one drug for one target (a "magic bullet"), the hunt is on for the combination of various drugs (a "magic shotgun") that will be beneficial for multiple targets.[42]

What is the best defense against multiple hits? I have coined the phrase **"multiple shields."** The good news is that you already have these shields; the challenge lies in keeping them healthy.

THE STORY OF A MAN WITH PARKINSON'S DISEASE

In 1901 a boy was born on the Lower East Side of Manhattan to immigrant parents. The boy's father owned a delicatessen. The family always had meat on the table. In fact, the daily fare revolved around meat and potatoes.

As the boy grew up, he became "a fat kid." When he was fourteen, his mother died. Without her love and guidance his teenage years were marked by living in the streets. He became a street fighter. Blows to the head were an almost daily occurrence.

When he was a teenager, he learned how to drive cars and trucks. Within a few years he landed a job as a New York City bus driver. The job was physically and emotionally stressful; it also involved long hours of sitting. Unfortunately, he never liked to take walks in his free time.

He married in the early 1920s. He and his wife had six children. Tragically, four of them died during the hard times of the Great Depression.

He did not contract the flu during the 1919 influenza epidemic but he came down with a severe illness, possibly a virus, in 1924. His wife was told to make preparations for his funeral. Miraculously, he beat the odds and survived.

In 1944 his wife died. And so, at the age of 43, he was a single parent to his two teenage children.

It was around this time that he began to develop health problems. He had trouble sleeping. He became constipated. He developed severe low back pain. Of course, each of these was attributed to his difficult life in an age when high levels of stress were the norm.

His job as a bus driver was good but he needed to make extra money. So, he spent extra hours in the depot repairing buses. Breathing in exhaust fumes from the buses that exited the depot was "just part of the job." He often worked nights; his sleep patterns continued to worsen.

By the mid-1950s, still obese, he became a borderline diabetic. He also noticed a slight tremor in his hands and remembered that several of his aunts, uncles, and cousins had "the shakes" too. In 1960 he began to have trouble steering the bus. His supervisor at the bus company told him that he needed to see the company doctor. That was when he was given the diagnosis of Parkinson's Disease and was forced into early retirement.

Until his death in 1986, he was plagued by tremors, poor balance, falls, severe constipation, difficulty urinating, excessive perspiration, difficulty swallowing, and medication-related problems. Once a powerful man, he weighed only 70 pounds at his death.

That man was my grandfather.

When I was a child, I wished that I could invent a time machine. I would travel back in time to take care of my grandfather when he was growing up. Maybe I would have been able to somehow slow down his Parkinson's Disease… but how?

My lifelong interest in PD led me to become a Doctor of Physical Therapy. Over my career I have read everything I could about PD. After decades of pouring through the literature, I began to understand the possible risk factors that lead to, and worsen, PD.

We can make some educated guesses about what may have contributed to my grandfather's Parkinson's Disease—his "multiple hits:"

> family history of tremors ("the shakes");

> poor diet (predominantly "meat and potatoes");

> obesity and borderline diabetes ("fat kid;" obese adult);

> head trauma (street fighter as a teenager);

➢ infection (life-threatening illness in the 1920s);

➢ lack of aerobic exercise (rarely walked, preferred to drive);

➢ emotional stress (deaths of his mother, four children, and his wife; financial worries; single father);

➢ poor sleep (difficulty sleeping; also worked night shifts);

➢ exposure to toxins and pollutants (exhaust fumes from buses);

➢ and of course, aging.

I never figured out how to invent my time machine. But I hope my childish dream of slowing down Parkinson's Disease will come true.

2

Our Multiple Shields

Our bodies have evolved to have multiple shields against the hits that we must endure. In this chapter we are going to take a tour of these defenses. We will try to follow a straight path, but we may have to occasionally backtrack to mention how one shield interacts synergistically with another.

Although our multiple shields have amazing protective properties, they are actually "two-faced," like the Roman god Janus. Just as he represented duality—looking to the past and to the future—our shields can either protect us or they can harm us. This is because each shield has an optimal range of its protective capabilities. Problems begin when their defenses are insufficient, or are excessive. Moreover, because of the normal synergy between shields, dysfunction in one shield can trigger dysfunction elsewhere.

PROCESSES:
HELPFUL AND HARMFUL

There are processes that have evolved to protect us. One of them is the reaction known as *inflammation*. To illustrate: let's say you suffer a fall and land on your knees. If it is bad enough, the trauma will lead to swollen, painful joints. The swelling and pain are signs that the body is trying to protect your knees: the buildup of fluids is the initiation of the healing process, and the pain serves as a reminder to avoid stressing the joints any further. The warmth that accompanies the swelling tells us that there is an increase in the chemical activity within your joints; this can also be seen by redness of the skin. As you heal, the inflammatory response will progress through its normal healing stages and will eventually subside. However, if the inflammatory response does not subside, it can become chronic; it can also have negative effects on other body parts.

There is another type of inflammation that is not so easy to visualize. It is called *neuroinflammation*—the reaction of the nervous system to injuries, infections, poor nutrition, disease, or toxins. Initially protective, neuroinflammation can be very dangerous. One of the hallmarks of PD is chronic, unchecked neuroinflammation.

Another type of process that is also "two-faced" is the growth of our bodies. Usually we weigh about six or seven pounds at birth. But within the first year our weight and height is multiplied; by the teenage years we approach normal adult size. One process that is responsible for this growth is abbreviated mTOR (for *mammalian Target of Rapamycin*). The mTOR pathway is partially fueled by what we eat, which stimulates growth factors. However, as we get older, the mTOR pathway can turn against us. For example: mTOR can trigger the wrong types of cell growth (such as cancer cells); mTOR can add to neuroinflammation; mTOR can also upset the normal functioning of healthy cells. Excessive mTOR activity is implicated in PD.[43]

Under normal circumstances, there are many other processes that keep us healthy. But they can become unbalanced in PD.[44] One is the maintenance of optimal amounts of calcium in and out of cells. But abnormalities of alpha-synuclein can disrupt this critically important process.[45] Another process involves the immune system, which protects against invading pathogens. Unfortunately, it sometimes turns on us, creating autoimmune diseases. Others processes involve maintaining the proper levels of signals that are transmitted within cells, and between cells.

OUR OUTERMOST SHIELD: THE SKIN AND MUCOUS MEMBRANES

We are covered by skin, our outermost barrier. There are several necessary openings in this layer, such as the nostrils and mouth. These openings allow us to breathe air and to ingest nutrients, respectively. But in doing so, the outside world is thus allowed to communicate with our inside world.

Even though our respiratory and digestive systems have their own defense mechanisms, they may not be effective enough to protect us from PD-inducing agents. Some nerve toxins can pass through the nasal passages and eventually wind up in the brain[46] where they trigger the production and spread of misfolded versions of alpha-synuclein.[47] As we will discuss later, there are toxins in our food supply; consumption of these chemicals may induce illness. Moreover, an unhealthy diet can alter the normal workings of our digestive tract, another amazing shield.

Here is an example of how the breakdown of shields leads to an abnormality in another shield: people with PD have a higher risk of developing a type of skin cancer called melanoma. Various theories have been proposed that link the misfolded protein alpha-synuclein to melanoma.[48]

THE SKULL

The brain is protected by a helmet-like structure, the skull. Usually the skull does an excellent job of protecting the brain if we suffer a minor blow to the head. However, repeated blows to the head, or severe head trauma, overwhelm the protective capabilities of this shield. But the damage does not stop in the brain: other shields far away from the head (such as the digestive tract) also become dysfunctional.

THE BLOOD-BRAIN BARRIER: LIKE A MEDIEVAL CASTLE WITH MANY LAYERS OF PROTECTION

Our brain cells have their own multiple shields. They are protected by the Blood-Brain Barrier (BBB). If it is healthy, it protects us from many of the disease-causing agents that we encounter during our lifetimes. The BBB allows the entry of healthy molecules; it also blocks harmful substances.

One of the world's foremost authorities on the BBB is Dr. Berislav Zlokovic. He has pioneered the idea that an unhealthy BBB is strongly implicated in PD,[49] as well as in other neurodegenerative conditions.[50] Breakdown of the BBB usually precedes PD.[51]

The BBB is comprised of over 400 miles of blood vessels; each of our 100 billion nerve cells (also known as *neurons*) has its own capillary.[52] It is important to keep in mind that what is unhealthy for our hearts and blood vessels (such as hypertension[53]) is also unhealthy for the BBB, and therefore, the brain.[54] In addition to blood vessels, the BBB is comprised of cells called astrocytes and pericytes, which regulate the nutrition, waste disposal, and overall health of neurons. Other types of cells, called microglia, are the immune soldiers of the BBB.

To better understand how this barrier works, we can compare it to another type of structure that evolved over many generations: the medieval castle.

Let's first describe the basic architecture. Medieval castles were constructed with two thoughts in mind: to safeguard the royal family (and their possessions), and to keep out their enemies. This was accomplished by building thick, high walls. Sometimes two walls were built: an outer wall and an inner wall. It was not uncommon for there to be a wide moat that surrounded the outer wall. Similarly, the BBB and the brain cells within are characterized by multiple layers of walls, or membranes. The "moats" of the BBB are filled with a liquid, called cerebral spinal fluid.

Castle walls were originally built of wood but evolved to more durable blocks of stone. However, despite the best of materials and designs, there were occasional design flaws that made some walls more vulnerable to attack, or simply to collapse. We also have design flaws: certain genetic mutations may leave us with inherent vulnerabilities.

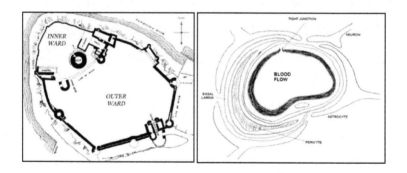

Castle defenses compared with your brain.

Left: Plan of the medieval castle in Pembroke, Wales.

Right: Cross-section of the Blood-Brain Barrier (BBB).

The multiple layers of defense of the BBB are similar to an inverted castle.

Trusted people were allowed to enter into the compound of the castle. In the brain, only certain molecules—needed for brain health, such as glucose—are normally allowed to enter through narrow openings of the BBB, called *tight junctions*. One common, tragic result of exposure to toxins, stress, trauma, infections, radiation, and certain diseases is that the tight junctions become wider than usual.[55] This allows the entry of potentially harmful substances into the brain.[56]

The outer walls of castles had openings; each type of opening had a specific shape. For example, there were vertical slits, which allowed archers to defend the castle. The vertical slits were for their vertical bows. But there were also horizontal slits, which were used by archers using horizontally-shaped crossbows. Circular openings were for defenders to shoot rifles. Similarly, the immune defenders of the BBB release a variety of molecules through specialized structures and pores.

A great deal of manpower was put into the defense of the walls. There were also a variety of defenders: besides the archers there were foot soldiers and the royal guards. There were also maintenance crews who continually inspected and repaired defects in the walls. A large labor force requires energy. The amount of mitochondria, the "powerhouses" of cells, is almost five times higher in the cells of the BBB, as compared to non-BBB regions of the brain.[57]

Just in case an attacker did actually get into the castle, he would often fall into a trap. These were designed to look like rooms. But once inside, the entry would be blocked, and he had no way to escape. This is not unlike the way our immune cells surround an invader and kill it. [58]

Moreover, if an attacker managed to get over to one of the spiral staircases of the castle, he would soon realize that the staircases were designed with "handedness:" the curves of the spiral favored right-handed defenders, who had ample room to swing their swords as they ran down the stairs. An attacker (probably also right-handed), would hit the wall when he tried to use his sword when he attempted to run up the stairs. The openings of the tight junctions also have "handedness:" only essential "right-handed" glucose is allowed to pass but another type of molecule, "left-handed" glucose, is blocked.[59]

Another method devised by the makers of the castle stair-cases was the construction of uneven steps. Those who lived in the castle adapted to the abnormal pattern of the steps, but any invaders would quickly trip, allowing the defenders to capture them. The BBB also has an irregularly-shaped wall, which "trips up" any pathogens that rub along the membrane. Once the pathogen is trapped, it is destroyed.

There was a rudimentary plumbing system in castles. There were pipes that were used for garbage disposal and latrines for human waste. The BBB also has an "efflux" system for getting rid of wastes. The brain possesses an intricate system of channels that widen while we sleep, facilitating brain fluids to wash away toxins. Moreover, the brain communicates with the gastrointestinal system via the vagus nerve—the longest nerve in the body. We will discuss the importance of the vagus nerve later in this chapter.

Within the castle walls there were a series of necessary structures: food storehouses, sleeping quarters, and the like. Each one had a valuable function for maintaining the daily life of the people who lived within the castle walls. Our structures are our brain cells, which produce chemicals (such as neurotransmitters) that allow us to function. Other important parts of the castle compound would be the farming areas, and the small fields for chickens and cows. These provided the basic but nutritious diet for those who lived within the castle walls.

Similarly, our cells require nutrition. The BBB allows entry for required nutrients.

And what of the people who lived within the castle walls? As we mentioned, there were the soldiers (like our immune system). There were also loyal workers who protected and maintained the castle, the royal family, and everything valuable inside the castle. Our loyal support is a healthy lifestyle (diet, sleep, exercise, and stress management). But who were the soldiers and the staff protecting and supporting? They took care of the royal family, and their valuables—the Crown Jewels. The aristocracy and their fortune kept medieval society functioning. They were, in a sense, the "currency" of their time. We also have types of currencies that are needed for the "transactions" of the brain: molecules that are produced within brain cells, which are needed for keeping us healthy. We will discuss the important cellular structures later.

But there were other types of people who lived within the castle. They were not loyal to the royal family. They were traitors, spies, hooligans, and other anti-social elements. They were locked up in the dungeons. They were feared because of their ability to incite others against the royal family. Our brains have a version of these types of people: free radicals. When they are generated in excess, they slowly destroy everything we want to protect. Our brains have a defense against free radicals: powerful anti-oxidants that are manufactured within and enhanced by a healthy lifestyle.

The immunity of the BBB is mediated by the microglia. But what happens when these protectors turn against us? Microglia play a critical role in neuroinflammation. Initially protective, the inflammatory response of the microglia can become toxic to dopamine-producing neurons.[60]

Castle fortresses were often under attack. The campaign to attack a castle was called a siege. There were short-term sieges, which caused temporary damage. We have several versions of short-term sieges: infections; acute stress; overheating; exhaustion. There were also long-term sieges, which over time, often caused the castle defenses to fail. Our long-term sieges are poor nutrition; prolonged stress; lack of exercise; poor sleep; or the combination of these factors. Aging can also be thought of as the accumulation of long-term wear and tear ("multiple hits"). These factors, coupled with our inherent vulnerabilities (genetic variations and mutations) lead to disease.

Sometimes dramatic, forceful attacks to the castle walls, such as those caused by battering rams, catapults, or trebuchets, caused a wall to collapse. Our versions of sudden, forceful breaks in the wall are traumatic brain injuries, or multiple concussions, which lead to severe consequences for our BBB.

Another type of increased pressure that the BBB must endure is hypertension. The increased pressure against the blood vessels causes additional openings, allowing the entry of various sized molecules—many of which are kept out under normal circumstances.[61]

Another unfortunate event that led to problems within the castle walls was when an excessive number of loyal soldiers were allowed entry. Even though they were trusted, their overcrowding upset the normal distribution of resources. Similarly, iron, a required nutrient, becomes dangerous if too much enters the brain.

Trickery was another method used by attackers. Instead of using force, they would masquerade as friendly soldiers in order to gain entry. Our BBBs are tricked by a buildup of harmful metals that resemble required elements. For example, manganese—a metal that is toxic when levels become excessive—enters via a mechanism that evolved for calcium entry.[62]

Some attackers were very clever. They smuggled themselves into the castle by going through the waste disposal pipes, which were rarely guarded. Most cases of PD are characterized by abnormal proteins and inflammatory cells that migrate from the gut to the brain through the vagus nerve.

What ultimately led to the downfall of the medieval castles? It was a new technology, which happened so fast and was so destructive that castle builders had little time to adapt: powerful cannons. Holes were blasted through castle walls, no matter how thick or well-protected. Similarly, we have not yet evolved protections against the wide range of toxins of our modern world.

PIGMENTED REGIONS AS SHIELDS AND REGULATORS

The BBB usually keeps "foreigners" out. But as we discussed, numerous toxins trick the BBB and gain entry. Once the toxins are inside, they may become trapped within specialized cells. These cells are pigmented—giving their regions a blue or black appearance. It is believed that the pigmented cells have a protective function: to grab onto contaminants. Pesticides, metals, and other toxic substances are captured by these pigmented cells, thus preventing their potentially hazardous spread.[63] When the level of contaminants reaches a critical level—exceeding the limit of the shield—a cascade of harmful reactions takes place. The pigmented neurons begin to degenerate. The toxins are released, free radical production is triggered, and neuroinflammation is worsened. The overload of toxic substances, over many years, tips the balance towards brain degeneration.[64]

One of these pigmented regions is called the *locus coeruleus*—the blue location. Another region is called the *substantia nigra*—the black substance. The locus coeruleus is where the neurotransmitter norepinephrine is produced. Norepinephrine helps us to wake up; it helps us to fall asleep; it allows us to react to stressful situations. Other functions of the locus coeruleus and norepinephrine are to regulate the reaction of the blood vessels of the BBB[65] and to suppress inflammation.[66] Therefore, the locus coeruleus is a shield of the BBB.[67] Degeneration of the locus coeruleus contributes significantly to Alzheimer's Disease[68] and PD.[69] Early pre-clinical PD signs, such as mood disorders and behavioral changes, can also be attributed to dysfunction of the locus coeruleus.[70]

The substantia nigra is where dopamine is produced. Just as degeneration of the locus coeruleus results in reduced norepinephrine production, degeneration of the substantia nigra leads to reduced dopamine production.[71] Besides the death of dopamine-producing cells, other vital structures (such as proteins that transport dopamine) also perish.[72] This is when the classical motor signs of PD appear. Unfortunately, degeneration in either the locus coeruleus or in the substantia nigra is detrimental to the other system—a perfect Janus-like example of one shield harming another.[73]

THE AUTONOMIC NERVOUS SYSTEM: THE AUTOMATIC CONTROLLER

There are several structures of the brain that do not have the protection of the BBB. These include the pineal gland and the hypothalamus. A healthy pineal gland is critical for sound sleep. A healthy hypothalamus regulates one's Autonomic Nervous System (ANS), which automatically maintains the heart, blood pressure, sleep, fatigue levels, hunger, thirst, sweating, and many other functions. Interestingly, stem cells—which give rise to new brain cells—also reside in an area that is not protected by the BBB.[74]

This normal lack of protection by the BBB is not a design flaw. It may have evolved to allow the easy entry of nutrients into these vital brain structures. But the lack of a shield makes the pineal gland, the hypothalamus, and other "non-BBB" brain areas especially vulnerable to toxic substances[75] and poor lifestyle choices.[76] If these "non-BBB" areas are not healthy, they can be a source of neuroinflammation that can spread to the rest of the brain.[77] Dysfunction of the pineal gland and the hypothalamus are responsible for sleep problems and other "non-motor" problems that precede the formal diagnosis of PD. Furthermore, it is feasible that an unhealthy environment would limit the ability of stem cells to transform into new brain cells.

The ANS can be thought of as an automatic series of sensors which instantly send messages to take corrective actions. Dr. David Goldstein, one of the world's foremost authorities on the ANS, has compared the actions of the ANS to the way that a thermostat works in your home heating system.[78] If you want the system to send up heat when the temperature drops below a certain point, let's say 65 degrees, you can adjust the set point to trigger the heating system at that temperature. Similarly, you can adjust the system to shut off at 70 degrees. In other words, the system will be activated at 65 and 70 degrees. This is the range at which you feel comfortable. But the human body has many "thermostat-like" mechanisms that maintain bodily functions (hunger, thirst, sleep, etc.). Each of them has a normal range—our "comfort zones."

A healthy ANS receives inputs and sends out responses to automatically guard us against dangerous changes to our comfort zones. Dysfunction of the ANS—such as what occurs in many cases of PD—leads to significant disability.[79]

The ANS can be broken down into four "zones:" the brain (including the hypothalamus and nearby structures); the sympathetic nervous system (which is generally responsible for stimulatory actions); the parasympathetic nervous system (which is generally responsible for calming actions); and the gut, which we will describe next.

THE INNER ECOSYSTEM: PART OF THE ANS, BUT DESERVES A SPECIAL WORD

The fourth part of the ANS is within the gut. The square footage of this region is roughly the size of a tennis court.

The gut is comprised of 100 million nerve cells. Plus, over 100 trillion microbes live there. Because of the huge number of nerves and microbes, the gut has two nicknames: "the second brain" and "the inner ecosystem."

When we have a balance of more beneficial microbes than harmful microbes, this shield is fortified and we enjoy good health. The openings of the intestine (called *tight junctions*, similar to what is found in the BBB) allow nutrients to be absorbed into the bloodstream. But if the gut is not healthy, the intestinal openings become abnormal and widen—allowing the entry of toxins and other unhealthy substances (including misfolded proteins) to enter the circulation. This is commonly referred to as "leaky gut;" the technical phrase is *increased intestinal permeability*. A recent study of nine people with PD demonstrated that all of them had increased intestinal permeability, as compared to normal, age-match controls.[80] Although the number of people studied was limited, this study is significant in that it also correlated the permeability of the gut with the absorption of alpha-synuclein—thus supporting Dr. Braak's hypothesis that the gut plays a major role in the development of PD. This is a very important line of research. Future studies, involving more people, will be useful.

THE SHIELDS WITHIN OUR CELLS

Let us now zoom in to discuss the shields of our brain cells. The outside of a cell, the cell membrane, is itself a shield. Fortified by the proper nutrients,[81] it keeps the structures of the cell enclosed. It allows only certain required molecules into the cell through specialized openings.

We can think of each cell as a protein factory. Just like any other type of factory, energy is required to keep everything running. The structures within cells that produce energy are the mitochondria; they are also responsible for other regulatory duties of the cell.[82] There are additional structures for the packaging of the proteins and for their transport within and out of the cells. Each of these cellular structures uses chemical messengers to communicate with each other, ensuring that the cell remains healthy.[83] Dysfunction of these other cell parts also contribute to PD.[84]

Using genetic material as a blueprint, the cell produces required proteins (such as alpha-synuclein) so that they are produced with the correct 3-dimensional folds, bends, and shapes. But sometimes proteins do not form correctly. They may be abnormally shaped, giving rise to misfolded proteins. Amazingly, we have evolved to have mechanisms that recognize misfolded proteins. These "bad proteins" are tagged for destruction by the cell's quality control systems:

> One of mechanisms these involves the *proteasome*, a submicroscopic shredding machine. Abnormally shaped proteins, tagged for recycling, go into one end of the barrel-shaped proteasome; amino acids, the building blocks for new proteins, come out at the other end.

> Another structure that destroys abnormally shaped proteins is the *lysosome*. The lysosome swallows up and destroys its target in a process referred to as autophagy ("self-eating"). Therefore, if a protein is misfolded—such as a misfolded version of alpha-synuclein—it should normally be destroyed.

> A third mechanism involves molecules that are produced in response to various stressors, such as a rise in body temperature. They are called *Heat Shock Proteins*, or HSPs. They are considered to be "chaperones" of proteins, helping with the correct folding of proteins. If a protein folds incorrectly,

HSPs have the critical role of "tagging" the proteins that need to be broken down. They also assist proteasomes and lysosomes in doing their jobs. In addition, HSPs can independently dissolve misfolded proteins.[85]

But what if the quality control mechanisms fail to work? This can occur due to genetics, poor diet, lack of sleep, insufficient exercise, exposure to toxins,[86] or other factors. There is evidence that the quality-control mechanisms communicate with each other.[87] If one fails, the other can increase its activity.[88] However, there is also evidence that a breakdown of one system may have adverse effects on the other.[89] It is also believed that aggregates, or clumps, of misfolded alpha-synuclein may be too large to fit into the opening of the tiny shredder, the proteasome. That leaves the lysosome to do the job of recycling.[90] Unfortunately, alpha-synuclein buildup is especially toxic to the lysosome.[91] If lysosomes become impaired, they cannot break down proteins. Therefore, both the proteasome and the lysosome fail to do their jobs. The resulting buildup of abnormal proteins becomes toxic to the mitochondria.[92] This tragic cascade of events leads to death of neurons and eventually, a disease such as PD.[93] There are several guiding principles for new drug development to treat PD. One of them is enhancing the health of cellular quality control mechanisms.[94] Another approach is preventing high levels of alpha-synuclein.[95]

THE VAGUS NERVE

We have made passing mention of the vagus nerve several times already. Let us discuss it in more detail. First of all, the name: "vagus" comes from the Latin word for wanderer, *vagare*. This nerve is a key structure of the ANS and connects the brain to distant organs, including the heart and gut. We have all experienced "butterflies," when nervous thoughts trigger feelings of unease in the stomach. We may also experience a skipped heartbeat. Also, if you are awakened from a deep sleep because of a stomach ache, thank the vagus nerve. In each of these scenarios the messages between the brain and the "second brain," the enteric nervous system, traveled through the vagus nerve.

Many lifestyle factors maintain the vagus nerve: exercise, stress relief, sleep, and a diet with healthy fats.[96] However, because of the winding path of the vagus nerve, sickness in one part of the body can lead to problems elsewhere. Unhealthy lifestyle factors (such as obesity, poor diet, lack of exercise, poor sleep, high levels of stress, exposure to toxins, and head injuries) diminish the protective shield of the vagus nerve.[97]

Abnormalities in the signals of the vagus nerve in the gut leads to a loss of function of dopamine in the brain.[98] Stem cells in the brain are also influenced by signals from the vagus nerve.[99] In an interesting experiment, researchers injected a type of toxin, classified as a "proteasome inhibitor," into the stomach of rats. As expected, the normal protective role of proteasomes was blocked. But the researchers also found that the toxin caused the clumping together of alpha-synuclein in the brain and degeneration in the vagus nerve.[100] Experiments such as this give tremendous support to Dr. Braak's theory of how the vagus nerve is a pathway for the spread of abnormal proteins.[101]

Dr. Kevin Tracey made an amazing breakthrough in the understanding of how the vagus nerve works. He found that in addition to conveying nerve signals, the vagus also plays a key role in inflammation.[102] As we discussed, PD is characterized by excessive neuroinflammation. One protein that is a powerful player in the inflammatory response is abbreviated HMGB1.[103] It also inhibits autophagy and accelerates the clumping together of alpha-synuclein.[104] Dr. Tracey has found that HMGB1 and other proteins that trigger inflammation can be inhibited by the actions of the vagus nerve.[105]

3

Genetics and Epigenetics

Having a close relative (such as a parent or sibling) with PD increases the risk of developing the disease.[106] A genetic study of over 600,000 people living in Iceland found that among relatives of people with adult-onset PD there was a definite pattern of increased risk. Siblings had an increased risk of between 4 and 10%; children had an increased risk of up to almost 8%; and nieces and nephews had an increased risk of approximately 2 to 4%.[107] The genetic risk may be higher for males than for females.[108]

For many years, PD was not considered to be a genetic disease. However, it is now known that quite a few mutations (also referred to as "susceptibility genes") are linked to the condition. This may explain why about 15-20% of people with PD have a family history of the disease.[109] However, none of the common PD genes have 100% "penetrance." What this means is that having a gene associated with PD may increase your risk, but it does not necessarily mean that you will get PD. This is why PD can run in families—but it also skips many relatives. As we will see, genes do not work alone.[110] There are multiple genes, combined with a variety of environmental insults, which lead to PD.[111] An often-repeated phrase is that "genetics loads the gun, but the environment pulls the trigger."[112]

EPIGENETICS

There is *genetics*—what you inherit—and then there is *epigenetics*—how genes are turned on and off by lifestyle and the environment. Epigenetics appears to play a key role in the development of neurodegenerative diseases.[113] The beneficial processes of a healthy lifestyle, coined "everyday epigenetics," may lower your risk of disease.[114] By improving your lifestyle you can maximize beneficial epigenetic processes and minimize the harmful ones. It is well established that inheriting a gene (or genes) for many diseases can be counteracted by maximizing health.[115]

Identical twins—both of whom share the same exact genes—have been studied. If PD were purely genetic, then if one of the twins develops PD, the other would

have a 100% risk of also developing PD. However, that
is not the case. The research illustrates the dynamics of
genetics versus epigenetics. There may be a higher risk
that both twins will get PD under the age of 50 (Young
Onset Parkinson's Disease). But Young Onset Parkinson's Disease is rare. Over the age of 50, no extraordinary
genetic risk was found.[116] Another study found that if
one identical twin develops PD, it is most likely due to
harmful environmental exposures that differed from the
"non-PD" twin.[117]

There are several molecular processes that can turn genes
on or off. One of these processes is called *methylation*.
During methylation, a specific molecule (methyl) connects to a genetic structure, thus influencing the expression of a gene or genes. The benefits of methylation are
linked to a healthy diet, exercise, avoidance of obesity,
and other lifestyle factors.[118] More research is needed to
explain the complexities of epigenetics regarding PD;
however, preliminary studies show that PD involves abnormalities in methylation.[119]

MicroRNAs, small molecules of genetic material, function to activate or deactivate genes. Several microRNAs
are related to PD.[120] MicroRNAs are influenced by our
multiple shields: diet,[121] exercise,[122] sleep,[123] and stress

management.[124] Unhealthy lifestyles result in alterations in levels of microRNAs.[125]

GENES LINKED TO PD

LRRK2: People with PD who have this mutation tend to decline slower than others with PD who have different mutations.[126] One of the common PD mutations is in a gene that produces, or *encodes*, a protein called *leucine-rich repeat kinase 2* (abbreviated as LRRK2). Believed to be a "master regulator," LRRK2 keeps cells functioning normally.[127] A mutated form of LRRK2 is known as G2019S. Having this mutated version increases the risk of developing PD and may also contribute to Alzheimer's Disease.[128] This is due to the detrimental effect that LRRK2 mutations have on autophagy, one of the cellular shields that breaks down and recycles abnormal proteins.[129] The membranes of lysosomes are also negatively affected by a LRRK2 mutation.[130] Abnormalities of LRRK2 may also increase inflammation of the nervous system.[131] Let us explore the penetrance of this mutated gene among carriers:[132]

Age of LRRK2 G2019S carrier	Percentage of carriers who develop PD	Percentage of carriers who *do not* develop PD
60 years old	15%	85%
70 years old	21%	79%
80 years old	32%	68%

As we can see, the majority of LRRK2 G2019S carriers do not develop PD, even with advanced age. Why do some LRRK2 G2019S carriers develop PD while others do not? Various types of genetic and epigenetic studies have begun to unravel this puzzle. Evidently, the combination of genes and lifestyle/environment makes the difference between health and disease. For example, some researchers have identified pesticide exposure[133] as a culprit for triggering PD in carriers of this mutation.

SNCA: The SNCA gene encodes alpha-synuclein, the protein that plays a role in the maintenance of cell membranes, release of neurotransmitters, and other vital functions. Mutations in this gene can result in the overproduction and/or accumulation of misfolded versions of alpha-synuclein.[134] Although having certain mutations of this gene are associated with an earlier age of onset of PD, they are *not* linked to how severe a case of

PD will be.[135] This suggests that epigenetic factors play an important role in long-term outcomes.

PARK7: PARK7 encodes the protein DJ-1. This protein has numerous shield-related functions: it regulates autophagy;[136] it binds to toxic metals, thus preventing damaging effects;[137] it protects cells from free-radical damage.[138] Mutations in DJ-1 result in a loss of these protective functions.[139]

PINK1: PTEN-induced putative kinase 1, or PINK1, is a gene that encodes an enzyme that protects the "powerhouses" of cells, the mitochondria. PINK1 mutations create vulnerabilities in mitochondria and result in a type of Young Onset Parkinson's Disease.[140]

Parkin: Mutations in the Parkin gene initiate a cascade of abnormal cellular processes, such as the dysregulation of DJ-1 and PINK1.[141] Mutations also inhibit the ability of proteasomes to breakdown misfolded proteins.[142]

HLA-DRB1: Human Leukocyte Antigen (HLA) genes produce proteins that regulate the immune system; DRB-1 refers to a specific subset of these genes. HLA-DRB1 mutations are associated with autoimmune diseases as well as PD. There is a growing recognition of the role of autoimmunity in PD.[143]

BDNF: Brain-Derived Neurotrophic Factor (BDNF) is beneficial molecule for the nervous system. Mutations in the gene for BDNF reduce the viability of this critical substance.[144] Mutations are not only linked to PD, but they may also lower the age at which one develops PD.[145]

MAPT: Deep within our cells are proteins that stabilize cellular structures; others create pipelines for the transport of molecules within cells. Some of these stabilizing proteins are called microtubules. A mutation in microtubule-associated protein *tau* (MAPT) can result in a collapse of the cellular framework and transport mechanisms. MAPT mutations are also associated with Alzheimer's Disease, PD, and Progressive Supranuclear Palsy (a "Parkinson's Plus" disease).[146]

APOE4: There is a gene that encodes a protein needed for cholesterol metabolism in the nervous system. It is called apolipoprotein E (APOE4). Mutations in APOE4 are associated with vascular disease in the brain, as well as with Alzheimer's and PD.[147]

GBA: This gene encodes an enzyme, glucocerebrosidase. The function of this enzyme is to break down a molecule called glucocerebroside into glucose and ceramide, a fat. A defect in the GBA gene may result in a loss of the normal "housekeeping" duties of cells: instead of glucocerebroside being broken down, it become "stored." This leads to what is referred to as a *storage disease*. Gaucher Disease is one such storage disease. Having Gaucher Disease increases the risk of developing PD by five-fold. This is probably due to the accumulation of glucocerebroside within nerve cells, which also triggers the aggregation[148] and spread[149] of alpha-synuclein.

ATP13A2: Mutations in this gene cause another type of a storage disease, linked to a rare Young Onset Parkinson's Disease.[150]

It is important to note that other genes may also play a role in the risk of developing PD. Over 900 PD associated genes have been identified so far.[151] They generally fall into the following shield-related categories:

➢ genes that encode antioxidants;[152]

➢ genes that encode repair of damaged cell components;[153]

➢ genes that encode cellular functioning;[154]

➢ genes that encode proteins that are part of the mitochondrial "machinery," to produce energy;[155]

> ➤ genes that encode neurogenesis;[156]

> ➤ genes that encode immune reactions in the gut;[157]

> ➤ genes that encode lysosomes[158] and proteasomes,[159] both of which degrade abnormal proteins.

DOCUMENTING THE MEDICAL HISTORY OF YOUR FAMILY

Having a family history of *any* type of tremor-related disease is associated with an elevated risk of developing PD.[160] The tremor of PD is usually a *resting* tremor—the affected body part will shake even if the patient is sitting quietly. By comparison, people who have a tremor while moving, such as reaching for a cup of water, are said to have an *action* tremor. This is usually the case in Essential Tremor. However, there may be an association between the two types of tremor. Some people with PD also have action tremors, and some people with Essential Tremor also have resting tremors. Suggestive of a common link, people with Essential Tremor have an increased risk of developing PD.[161]

Mood disorders, such as depression or bipolar disorder, also pose an increased risk of developing PD. [162]

However, this connection is somewhat cloudy. Is a depressed person actually exhibiting pre-clinical PD? Is it related to alterations in neurotransmitters? Is it the medications used to treat these disorders that trigger PD?

A family history of Alzheimer's Disease is also significant. It has been found that several genes associated with Alzheimer's have a connection with PD.[163] There is considerable overlap between the two diseases.[164]

Crohn's Disease, a chronic inflammatory condition of the digestive tract, also shares a genetic link with PD.[165]

It is a good idea to document the medical history of your family. Make special note of the following:

> If you have a family history of any type of tremor, mood disorder, autoimmune disease, storage disease (such as Gaucher), or neurodegenerative disease;

> If your relative was diagnosed with PD or another neurological condition, document the age of diagnosis (if known) as well as the age of death;

> Your relative's occupation. Was there exposure to toxins, such as pesticides?

> ➤ Any other medical conditions. As we will see in upcoming chapters, some medical conditions may be associated with PD.

YOUR ACTION PLAN

☞   Document the medical history of your family using *My Family Health Portrait* (A Tool from the Surgeon General):

https://familyhistory.hhs.gov/fhh-web/home.action

☞   Parkinson's Disease Mutation Database:

http://www.thepi.org/parkinson-s-disease-mutation-database/

☞   Genetics and PD:

http://ghr.nlm.nih.gov/condition/parkinson-disease

☞   Locating a certified Genetic Counselor:

http://nsgc.org/p/cm/ld/fid=164

National Gaucher Foundation, Inc.:

http://www.gaucherdisease.org/

4

Diet

Before we discuss the details of a personalized diet, allow me to tell you the story of one of my patients with PD.

Frieda (not her real name) lived alone. Her husband died many years ago. She did not have any children or any close friends. She had been taking L-Dopa for about two years. Most of her food was delivered from the local deli. Her meals were generally turkey or roast beef sandwiches, buttered rolls, and cookies. Her favorites drinks were sodas.

Frieda was not doing well. Her movements continued to worsen. Getting out of bed was difficult and she began to fall. The physical act of eating became harder and harder.

My physical therapy evaluation (in her home) revealed that she had poor posture, weakness, limited mobility in her arms and legs, and poor balance. Frieda was very frail and underweight. She could only walk from room to room, holding onto furniture for support. She had difficulty speaking, and she drooled (which usually means difficulty with swallowing). Frieda allowed me to open her refrigerator. It was almost empty. In other words, Frieda was not cared for. Her lack of proper nutrition was obvious. And her high consumption of protein probably interfered with her body's abilty to absorb L-Dopa. This could explain the worsening of her movement skills: it was if she did not have any medication in her system. She had difficulty grasping a fork and raising food to her mouth. Frieda also complained that her dentures hurt; chewing and swallowing food was problematic.

Moreover, her abdomen was bloated. She moved her bowels only once a week.

I discussed the case with her neurologist. Ultimately, Frieda was referred to the following members of the healthcare team:

1. A dietician, who worked out meal plans. She took into account the amount, and timing, of protein intake so as to maximize Frieda's L-Dopa absorption. The dietician also learned that Frieda had

food allergies. The meal plans maximized tasty, allergy-free, nutritionally-dense meals;

2. A dentist, who made new, comfortable dentures;

3. A Speech Pathologist, who helped Frieda improve her ability to chew and to swallow;

4. A gastroenterologist, who found that Frieda's constipation was worsened by SIBO: Small Intestinal Bacterial Overgrowth. With treatment, her bowel movements improved;

5. A home care agency, which provided a home attendant who assisted with food shopping, meal preparation, and feeding.

As you can see, it took a small army of people to personalize Frieda's ability to eat (and to absorb her food and medications). Within a few weeks the exercises that I gave Frieda resulted in improvements in strength and mobility. She gained weight. Overall, was able to enjoy an improved quality of life.

Any discussion of the personalization of "diet" is incomplete if the other aspects of food purchasing, storage, preparation, eating, digestion and elimination are not taken into account.

Now, let's begin our discussion of food.

We all want to enjoy meals that are nutritious. But what constitutes "nutritious" in the context of PD? The accelerated loss of dopamine and other neurotransmitters are hallmarks of PD; diets that minimize their loss (beyond normal aging) would be ideal. Studies suggest that certain foods and dietary patterns may promote PD by weakening our protective shields. Interestingly, a dietary study of newly diagnosed people with PD found that their normal food intake was characterized by highly refined carbohydrates (in other words, processed foods). They also had extremely low amounts of protein and vitamin/mineral-rich foods.[166]

Other foods and dietary patterns may protect against PD.[167] **For someone with PD, a diet high in fruits and vegetables may be the difference between a slow progression, versus a rapid deterioration.**[168]

BASIC NUTRITIONAL RULE #1: OUR GENES, CELLS, AND NEUROTRANSMITTERS REQUIRE A HEALTHY DIET.

It has been known for many years that the cellular damage caused by a poor diet mimics the damaging effects of radiation.[169] As we mentioned in the last chapter, our genes need certain nutrients for epigenetic processes to take place. When epigenetic processes do not function properly (such as too little or too much methylation) diseases such as PD can occur.

The shields within our cells function best when we have adequate levels of nutrients. For example, lysosomes (which break down and recycle unneeded substances in cells) require Vitamin C,[170] Vitamin D,[171] and other vital nutrients, such as minerals.[172]

Neurotransmitters are produced when precursor amino acids are available.[173] Serotonin requires the precursor tryptophan; dopamine, epinephrine and norepinephrine require the precursor tyrosine; and acetylcholine requires the precursor choline. Eating a predominantly plant-based diet,[174] supplemented with small amounts of animal products, provide these precursors for neuro-transmitter production.

BASIC NUTRITIONAL RULE #2: THERE IS A NATURAL BALANCE BETWEEN PRO-OXIDANTS AND ANTIOXIDANTS.

We need oxygen to survive. As a result of using oxygen, our bodies produce molecules called free radicals. They are needed for chemical reactions in the body; however, excessive levels of free radical production can harm tissues and are linked to a host of diseases, including PD. Some substances, called *pro-oxidants*, trigger the increased production of free radicals. Iron is an example of a pro-oxidant. But we have evolved to keep the free radicals in balance, by means of *antioxidants*. A diet rich in antioxidants, and in factors that are needed for the body to produce antioxidants naturally, may reduce the risk of PD.[175] For example, Vitamin C is an antioxidant and also has other key anti-PD roles. It is needed for epigenetic regulation;[176] for the manufacture of neurotransmitters, for regulating the immune system, and for working together with other vitamins.[177]

BASIC NUTRITIONAL RULE #3: EAT FOODS THAT REDUCE NEURO-INFLAMMATION.

Neuroinflammation, the chronic inflammation of the nervous system, is another characteristic of PD. Inflammation appears to be a key player in the triggering of iron-related inbalance in the brains of patients with PD.[178] Interventions that decrease inflammation are primary goals of Parkinson's researchers.[179] Anti-inflammatory foods may be beneficial in the treatment of PD.[180]

BASIC NUTRITIONAL RULE#4: EAT FOODS THAT INHIBIT THE *MTOR* PATHWAY AND ENHANCE THE PATHWAYS THAT BREAK DOWN ABNORMAL PROTEINS.

The two structures within our cells that break down abnormal proteins are the lysosome and the proteasome. Certain foods can stimulate them, while other foods can inhibit them.

The mTOR pathway leads to abnormal cellular functioning. It is linked to diabetes, hypertension, autoimmune diseases, cancer, and neurodegenerative diseases, such as PD.[181] When mTOR pathways are activated, the activity of the lysosome (called *autophagy*) is diminished. As a result, waste products tend to build up in cells; this leads to neurodegeneration. The mTOR pathway also drives the clumping together of alpha-synuclein.[182] Fortunately, the mTOR pathway can be somewhat inhibited and autophagy can be enhanced with the proper diet.[183]

BASIC NUTRITIONAL RULE #5: ENHANCE YOUR INNER ECO-SYSTEM PROTECTION SYSTEM.

A healthy diet promotes a healthy gut, also known as our "second brain." The types of beneficial versus harmful microbes are strongly related to our diets. It is postulated that a plant-based diet triggers a cascade of helpful reactions in our gut bacteria, thus protecting the nervous system.[184] About 95% of the body's serotonin is found in the gastrointestinal tract. Serotonin plays multiple key roles in maintaining the digestive system, the Autonomic Nervous System, and the "brain-gut connection."[185] Almost all patients with PD develop gut dysfunction[186] and intestinal inflammation.[187] Keeping the gut healthy is highly neuroprotective. Amazingly, switching to a healthy diet can change the composition of gut bacteria to a more favorable profile *within 24 hours.*[188]

BASIC NUTRITIONAL RULE #6: EAT FOODS THAT ARE GOOD FOR THE BLOOD-BRAIN BARRIER (BBB).

The BBB is a primary shield for the brain. High fat and high calorie diets are nutrient depleted. They are bad for the BBB[189] and are linked to PD. Plant-based diets are low in calories and are nutrient-dense. They are good for the BBB and the entire nervous system.

BASIC NUTRITIONAL RULE #7: EAT FOODS THAT CHELATE (BIND TO) METALS.

PD is linked to abnormal levels of iron, zinc, lead, mercury, aluminum, manganese, and copper. These metals can trigger excessive levels of free radicals. Certain nutrients have the capacity to bind to these metals to lower their levels of toxicity.

BASIC NUTRITIONAL RULE #8: EAT FOODS THAT INHIBIT THE MISFOLDING AND CLUMPING OF ALPHA-SYNUCLEIN.

A wide range of compounds found in foods may inhibit the misfolding and aggregation of alpha-synuclein. Furthermore, when the pH, or acidity, of our body fluids is too low it is known as *metabolic acidosis*. This acidic environment is detrimental to the nervous system;[190] it also promotes the misfolding of proteins. [191] Indeed, the clumping together of alpha-synuclein increases dramatically in an acidic cellular environment.[192] A plant-based diet reverses metabolic acidosis.[193]

FOODS AND DIETARY PATTERNS THAT MAY ACCELERATE PD

SAD: The Standard American Diet

Pizza. Cheeseburgers. French fries. Milkshakes. Donuts. Soda. These fast foods are part of the common fare of the Western Diet, also known as the Standard American Diet ("SAD"). SAD is characterized by refined carbohydrates (sugary foods), salty foods, and foods that are high in trans-fats and saturated fats.

It is important to remember that fat *per se* is not dangerous. In fact, fat is needed by every cell in the human body. Cholesterol, a type of fat, is concentrated in the brain and is vital for proper brain functioning. The BBB has a natural ability to process cholesterol. But this process is altered by an unhealthy diet, such as SAD.[194]

Trans-fats are fats that have been artificially altered to make them less likely to spoil. They are commonly found in fried foods, cookies, and pastries. Trans-fats may be the leading cause of heart disease[195] and they also contribute to other diseases, such as neurodegeneration.[196]

A diet high in saturated fat—the type of fat found in animal meat and high fat dairy—is linked to a greater risk of PD.[197] A lifelong, high-fat diet can be considered to be a risk factor for developing PD.[198] There are many reasons why our multiple shields are harmed by a high fat diet:

> ➢ it not only leads to obesity, but also to a loss of dopamine;[199]

➢ it lowers the threshold for the susceptibility to toxins;[200]

➢ it upsets the balance of the Autonomic Nervous System;[201]

➢ it alters methylation patterns, causing dysfunction of the hypothalamus;[202]

➢ it leads to metabolic acidosis,[203] which facilitates the abnormal folding of proteins;

➢ it inhibits autophagy;[204]

➢ it causes dysregulation of the proteasome system;[205]

➢ it triggers brain inflammation;[206]

➢ it lowers levels of a repair molecule, hepatocyte growth factor;[207]

➢ it impairs the BBB and damages the hippocampus, resulting in a loss in cognition;[208]

> ➢ it weakens the normally protective activity of the DJ-1 protein.[209] This is of critical importance, as DJ-1 is an inhibitor of alpha-synuclein.[210] Similarly, a high-fat diet negatively alters the functioning of another PD-related gene, Parkin.[211]

Fried foods pose yet another danger. The frying of oils causes the production of two related molecules called acrolein and acrylamide.[212] These are powerful neurotoxins—chemicals that destroy nerve cells.[213] Acrolein and acrylamide are found in high levels in the brains of people with neurodegenerative diseases.[214]

Highly processed breads and desserts contain aluminum,[215] which over the long-term leads to cognitive impairment.[216] Refined carbohydrates also contribute to neurodegeneration.[217]

High levels of salt in the diet have the potential to disrupt the balance of the Autonomic Nervous System,[218] alter the levels of antioxidants in the brain, and contribute to memory loss.[219] Moreover, the risk of autoimmune diseases is raised by consuming excessive salt. In particular, levels of specific immune cells (called T helper 17), become stimulated by a salty diet.[220] It has been proposed that PD is actually an autoimmune disease: T helper 17 cells react to alpha-synuclein.[221]

Advanced glycation end-products (AGEs)

Advanced glycation end-products, aptly abbreviated "AGEs," are compounds that are formed during the heating of sugars and proteins. Excessive levels of AGEs are associated with aging and many diseases, including PD.[222] The misfolding of alpha-synuclein can be induced by AGEs.[223] Moreover, AGEs lower levels of a powerful antioxidant, glutathione.[224] They are also inflammatory[225] and can trigger neuroinflammation in neurons.[226] The highest levels of AGEs are found in barbecued meats, pizza, cheeses, fried foods,[227] pastries, and cookies.[228]

High iron foods

Iron is a critical nutrient. Low levels of iron can result in anemia. Iron-deficiency anemia is a risk factor for the development of PD, especially in females.[229] Levels of iron are usually well-regulated in the brain. But if this regulatory process fails, excessive iron can accumulate.[230]

There are two main types of iron in our diets. One is referred to as "heme" iron, found especially in red meat; the other is "non-heme" iron, found in iron fortified foods, such as breakfast cereals, bread, and iron supplements. A high dietary level of iron increases the risk of PD.[231] Iron becomes concentrated in the substantia nigra.[232] If the high level of iron is combined with a high level of manganese (found in cereals), the risk of PD is doubled.[233] It is prudent to limit the intake of breakfast cereals and bread, both of which have high levels of non-heme iron and manganese.

High levels of iron accelerate oxidation in the brain and results in a loss of dopamine-producing cells. Animal studies have demonstrated that excessive iron consumption leads to "iron overload" and PD.[234] Iron supplements should only be taken when medically necessary.[235]

When increased levels of iron are combined with exposure to the pesticide paraquat, the neurodegeneration of PD is accelerated.[236]

Meat

There are numerous reasons why high levels of meat consumption may worsen PD, as meat contains high levels of:

> ➢ heme iron;

➤ the amino acid leucine, which triggers the mTOR pathway;[237]

➤ cholesterol and unhealthy saturated fats, both of which have been linked to PD;[238]

➤ contaminants: veterinary drugs (such as antibiotics), metals, and pesticides (as per an audit by the United States Department of Agriculture's Attorney General);[239]

➤ endotoxins (especially in ground beef): they are components of bacteria (such as *E. coli*). Endotoxins have been suggested as a culprit in the cause of PD, possibly through the disruption of the balance of healthy gut bacteria.[240]

We already mentioned that when meat is cooked at high temperatures (such as at a barbeque), AGEs are formed. In addition, multiple neurotoxins are produced. Two of these toxins, harman and norharman, have a chemical structure similar to a known PD-inducing chemical, MPTP. Levels of both of these toxins are found in high levels in people with PD[241] and Essential Tremor.[242] Fortunately, the levels of harman and norharman can be reduced significantly by seasoning the meat with red pepper,[243] black pepper,[244] or other spices that have high levels of antioxidants.[245]

However, it important to keep in mind that meat does have important health benefits, *when eaten in small portions*. We will discuss this later.

Milk and cheese

Numerous studies have consistently shown that the consumption of milk and cheese increases the risk of PD. It has been estimated that one's risk of developing PD increases by 17% for each 200 ml (7 ounce) glass of milk per day, and 13% for each 10 grams (only 1/3 of an ounce!) of cheese per day.[246] It may be that the safest dairy product to eat is yogurt (we will discuss this later).

There are numerous reasons as to why milk and cheese are linked to PD:

> ➤ There may be pesticide residues found in milk;[247]

> ➤ Casein, a milk protein, interferes with the body's natural balance of urate, a strong antioxidant;[248]

➢ Two components of casein can form toxic misfolded proteins,[249] similar to those found in type 2
diabetes,[250] Alzheimer's, and PD;[251]

➢ Whole milk is high in triglycerides, which impair
the BBB;

➢ Milk has a high glycemic index[252] (discussed later);

➢ Milk may contain radon, a radioactive gas;[253]

➢ Milk may contain a type of bacteria, *Mycobacterium paratuberculosis*. It can survive the pasteuri-
zation process.[254] It causes inflammation of the gut
and contributes to Crohn's Disease; it may also
trigger PD and worsen neurodegeneration;[255]

➢ Milk consumption fosters the growth of an extremely unhealthy gut organism, *bilophila
wadsworthia*. It causes increased intestinal permeability.[256] It is also one of the most common bacteria implicated in appendicitis.[257]

It is estimated that 70% of appendicitis cases are
related to a low-fiber diet and constipation.[258] The
appendix in humans has traditionally been considered to be a useless body part. However, it is now

believed that it serves as a storehouse for healthy gut bacteria; the appendix is part of the immunity system of the intestines.[259] The appendix also has high levels of alpha-synuclein. [260]

In summary, there may be a link between an unhealthy diet that includes milk, *bilophila wadsworthia*, an unhealthy appendix, increased intestinal permeability, and the spread of alpha-synuclein in the gut;

➢ Milk contains high levels of insulin-like growth factor (IGF). This substance developed over the generations of evolutionary history to aid in infant growth. However, once we outgrow the breast-feeding stage, milk ingestion can trigger the growth of other types of cells, such as fat cells. IGF is a strong trigger of the mTOR pathway.[261] This is detrimental to our cells, as mTOR inhibits autophagy;[262]

➢ Processed cheese is high in aluminum, a neurotoxin. [263] Cheese is made with the use of potassium alum, to bleach milk,[264] and aluminum phosphate, an emulsifying agent. Frozen pizza has especially high levels of aluminum. [265] Many cheeses are high in AGEs.[266]

Excessive alcohol consumption

Having one alcoholic or non-alcoholic drink per day is linked to a reduced risk of PD (discussed later). But high alcohol consumption causes alcohol-related brain damage. [267] Alcohol worsens neuroinflammation.[268]

When consumed in excess, alcohol is a neurotoxin and disrupts cellular shields. This leads to lower levels of dopamine production.[269] Moreover, alcoholics (and drug addicts) have lower levels of nerve receptors for dopamine. The number of receptors continues to decrease with chronic alcoholic abuse. This is probably due to aging, alcoholism itself, or other factors,[270] such as the poor nutritional status of alcoholics. [271] Chronic alcohol abuse decreases proteasome activity within cells.[272]

Foods high in omega-6 fatty acids

The membranes of brain cells contain *essential fatty acids*. They are called "essential" because they are required for the body; they can only be obtained from the proper diet. Fatty acids are further classified by their chemical structures, giving rise to the categories of "omega-3 fatty acids" and "omega-6 fatty acids." Sixty percent of the brain is composed of fats, primarily omega-3.[273]

Of the two, omega-3 fatty acids are generally deficient in the Western diet. Diets that have excessively high levels of omega-6 fatty acids are linked to cardiac disease, arthritis, and other inflammatory conditions—including PD.[274] Dopamine-producing neurons are especially vulnerable to low levels of omega-3 and high levels of omega-6 fatty acids.[275]

It has been discovered that ratios of omega-6/omega-3 fatty acids for minimizing diseases ranges between 2/1 to 5/1. A ratio of 4/1 is associated with an amazing 70% reduction in mortality.[276] This ratio is also associated with an improvement in BBB functions, improved sleep, lowered stress levels, and decreased dementia.[277] By comparison, the ratio of omega-6/omega-3 fatty acids in the Standard American Diet is approximately 16/1.

It is prudent to minimize consumption of foods that are high in omega-6 fatty acids, such as grapeseed oil, sunflower oil, corn oil, soybean oil, cottonseed oil, and margarine.[278]

High sugar intake

Chronically high levels of sugar consumption leads to elevated blood levels of insulin, which has been linked not only to diabetes and obesity ("diabesity"), but also to the onset of PD.[279] High glucose levels worsen the effects of high levels of iron, hastening the death of nerve cells.[280] A diet characterized by sugary foods is also high in AGEs.[281] When sugar molecules interact with proteins, the unwanted process of *glycation* takes place. Glycation has been shown to worsen the toxic reactions of alpha-synuclein, resulting in the death of dopamine-producing cells.[282]

Well water

Due to possible contamination from pesticides and other pollutants, well water as a source of one's drinking water has been linked to a high risk of developing PD. [283] If you do drink from well water, it is important to have your water tested to find out if it is contaminated.

FOODS AND DIETARY PATTERNS THAT MAY SLOW PD

Organic foods

The pesticides and toxins that permeate our food supply increase the risk of developing PD.[284] Organically grown food has significantly lower levels of contamination. Extensive testing was done on organic fruits and vegetables compared to conventionally grown produce. It was found that organically grown food has about 25% of the contaminant levels of non-organically grown food.[285]

In a fascinating study, 23 children (aged 3 to 11) who were switched to organically grown food showed a dramatic change in their urine samples: levels of pesticides disappeared. This change occurred in as little as 8 to 36 hours.[286]

Unfortunately, imported foods may contain higher levels of pesticides as compared to those regulated in the USA. In addition, imported foods may contain residues of pesticides that are banned in the USA.[287] The solution may be to eat only locally, organically grown fresh fruits and vegetables that are in season.

Small servings of lean, unprocessed, organic meat

A meal that includes a small serving of lean, unprocessed, organic meat provides factors that are neuropreventative. Many of them cannot readily be found in a vegan or vegetarian diet:

> ➢ zinc, needed for the production of metallothioneins, which are proteins that can chelate various toxic metals. Metallothioneins also inhibit the aggregation of alpha-synuclein, boost levels of antioxidants glutathione and Coenzyme Q10, and prevent iron accumulation.[288] Zinc is critical for the production of several neurotransmitters as well as for the immune system.[289] Zinc raises levels of hepatocyte growth factor, a repair molecule that is deficient in PD and many other diseases.[290] Zinc increases the activity of proteasomes, the tiny "shredders" within cells that shield against misfolded proteins.[291] Adequate levels of zinc in the diet may prevent PD;[292]

> ➢ selenium, needed for glutathione production[293] and for lowering levels of the toxic protein homocysteine[294] (discussed later in this chapter);

➤ cysteine. Not only does cysteine chelate metals,[295] but it is also needed for the production of metallothioneins and glutathione (discussed later in this chapter);

➤ tyrosine, needed for the production of neurotransmitters. Tyrosine is the precursor of dopamine, as well as norepinephrine and epinephrine;[296]

➤ glutamine, needed to block the absorption of toxins and bacteria through the intestines.[297] It also activates autophagy;[298]

➤ carnosine, which helps to protect the nervous system from neurodegenerative diseases[299] and protects against AGEs;[300]

➤ Vitamin B12, which lowers levels of homocysteine.[301]

Foods high in omega-3 fatty acids

There are many reasons why the proper levels of omega-3 fatty acids are anti-PD:

➤ Omega-3 fatty acids work via an epigenetic mechanism, resulting in proper levels of a gene that turns on the dopamine-producing system; [302]

➤ A diet rich in omega-3 fatty acids protects neurons from toxin-induced PD. Moreover, the dangers of chronic pesticide exposure are somewhat lessened by these protective fatty acids.[303] By comparison, high levels of omega-6 fatty acids appear to worsen one's reaction to air pollution and the negative effects of smoking;[304]

➤ Omega-3 fatty acids are a critical part of structures within cell membranes called *lipid rafts*. Their job is to assist with the transmission of signals in the cell. Researchers have found that alterations of lipid rafts is associated not only with neurodegeneration, but with a host of inflammatory conditions, as well as cancer; the addition of omega-3 fatty acids to a diet is thus preventative for many diseases.[305] People with PD have dysfunctional lipid rafts in PD, characterized by low levels of omega-3 fatty acids.[306] Mutations in the LRRK2 gene are associated with dysfunction of lipid rafts.[307] It is possible that the aggregation of alpha-synuclein is due to changes in lipid rafts;[308]

➢ Omega-3 fatty acids are not just found in cell membranes. They are also found in the membranes of vesicles that store, transport, and release neurotransmitters. A deficiency of omega-3 fatty acids disrupts the composition of these vesicle membranes, thus preventing the normal transmission of dopamine and other neurotransmitters;[309]

➢ Omega-3 fatty acids raise levels of neurotrophic factors in the brain;[310]

➢ Omega-3 fatty acids are anti-inflammatory.[311] This anti-inflammatory effect protects the gut and autonomic nervous system as well, via the vagus nerve;[312]

➢ Omega-3 fatty acids regulate the entry of glucose into the cells of the BBB. In an amazing study, the addition of omega-3 fatty acids shifted the amount of glucose transport from a deficiency of 23% to an enhancement of 35%—a total improvement of 57%, thus protecting the BBB;[313]

Fruits and vegetables have a naturally low omega 6/omega 3 fatty acid ratio. The following foods are richest in omega-3 fatty acids: flax seeds, salmon, sardines, beef, and soybeans.[314]

Fish

Wild Alaskan salmon has high levels of omega-3 fatty acids[315] and high levels of Vitamin D.[316] Fish oil improves the responsiveness of the vagus nerve.[317] Fish consumption also decreases the mTOR pathway.[318] But be aware of high mercury levels in fish. Wild Alaskan salmon may be the safest to eat in terms of lowest levels of mercury.[319] Interestingly, fish also contains high levels of selenium, which may mitigate the toxic effects of mercury.[320] In order to gain the immense benefits of fish while minimizing the risks of mercury exposure, it is recommended to consume 8 ounces of fish per week.[321]

Eggs

Egg consumption is linked to a lower risk of PD.[322] There are several possible reasons for this. Eggs have high levels of tyrosine, needed for the production of neurotransmitters.[323] Eggs are also rich sources of Vitamin D, choline, and methionine, needed for important epigenetic processes to occur.[324]

Mediterranean diets

The term "Mediterranean Diet" is a bit of a misnomer. There are actually quite a few variations of the diet, each of which arose independently in Spain, Italy, Greece, and in neighboring countries. Similar diets are the traditional Chinese and Japanese diets, giving rise to the term "Mediterrasian diet"—emphasizing the benefits of Mediterranean and Oriental diets. The Mediterrasian diet has been proposed to yield health benefits similar to caloric restriction. [325]

What each of them has in common is a predominantly plant-based diet, seasoned with olive oil, with limited amounts of whole grains, nuts, meat and fish.[326] The result is a healthy ratio of omega-6/omega-3 fatty acids. A Mediterranean diet lowers the expression of genes that trigger inflammation.[327]

A diet high in vegetables, fruits, and fish was associated with a lower risk of PD as compared to the standard Western diet.[328] These diets stimulate neurogenesis (the growth of new brain cells).[329] Other diets exist that are also plant-based and have numerous health benefits, such as DASH (Dietary Approach to Stop Hypertension).

But it is important to remember that a healthy diet must be a consistent lifestyle change, not just a short-term fad. People who adhere to a Mediterranean diet have lower odds of developing PD.[330]

Nitrates

Nitrates and nitrites are naturally occurring compounds; highest levels are found in spinach, beets, lettuce, and celery. When consumed, nitrates and nitrites are converted into nitric oxide, a neurotransmitter and potent dilator of blood vessels—thereby lowering blood pressure and improving exercise performance.[331]

Edible seaweeds

Edible seaweeds, such as spirulina and kelp, are sea algae. They are considered to be "complete proteins," as they provide all of the essential amino acids.[332] Seaweeds are also high in mannitol. Not only does mannitol penetrate the BBB, but it is also a powerful agent for preventing the aggregation of alpha-synuclein and for reducing its levels in the brain. This has been demonstrated not only in laboratory tests, but also in insects and mice that have an experimental version of PD.[333] Moreover, seaweeds contain compounds that can stimulate production of hepatocyte growth factor, which is neuroprotective.[334]

Fiber and fermented foods (includes yogurt and related products)

Another advantage of a mostly plant-based diet is the amount of fiber consumed. When fiber ferments in the colon, short-chain fatty acids (SCFA) are produced; SCFAs are anti-inflammatory.[335] This anti-inflammatory effect occurs not only in the gut, but also in the brain: in the BBB[336] and in the hypothalamus. The signals of the hypothalamus help to regulate weight loss that occurs with a healthy gut.[337]

Fiber acts as food for the healthy organisms that we consume, referred to as *probiotics*. Fiber is therefore a *prebiotic*. The combination (and synergistic effect) of prebiotics and probiotics is referred to as *synbiotics*.[338]

One type of prebiotic, inulin, is found in artichokes, chickory root, leeks, onions, garlic, bananas, and beets.[339]

Natto (fermented soybeans) has high levels of quinone, a compound that inhibits transglutaminase (the dangerous enzyme activated by gluten).[340]

Although milk consumption is strongly linked to PD, the fermentation of milk produces anti-PD substances. Fermented milk products are yogurt, buttermilk, kefir, sour cream, and acidophilus milk.

Probiotics prevent PD in a variety of ways:

➤ They promote a healthy gut by preventing increased intestinal permeability;[341]

➤ They inhibit harmful gut organisms, such as *bilophila wadsworthia*;[342]

➤ They inhibit the growth of *Streptococcus mutans*.[343] This dental organism can trigger the misfolding of proteins;[344]

➤ They exert a beneficial epigenetic effect;[345]

➤ They are anti-inflammatory;[346]

➤ They raise levels of Vitamin B12 and lower levels of homocysteine;[347]

> ➤ They raise levels of BDNF in the brain;[348]

> ➤ The consumption of probiotic-rich fermented milk products reduces the effects of stress in the midbrain.[349]

Water

Water is critical for life. Often overlooked in discussions of brain health, water intake is essential for maintaining normal fluid balances in the body. Dehydration is disruptive to the BBB.[350] As we will discuss, tea and coffee have been shown to be beneficial for brain health. But another reason why they are beneficial is that both require water.[351]

Even mild dehydration may lead to constipation.[352] This is to be avoided, as chronic and/or severe constipation is a common problem in PD.[353] Dehydration may contribute to the spread of misfolded proteins from the gut to the nervous system.[354]

An average sedentary male requires about 12 cups of water a day. An average sedentary female requires about 9 cups a day.[355] As activity levels rise, so does the need for additional fluid intake. But you do not have to gulp down so many glasses of water. Fortunately, a plant-based diet will automatically provide a generous amount of water. Most fruits and vegetables contain approximately 80-95% water.[356]

Foods high in B vitamins

Our cells depend on B vitamins for proper functioning. A deficiency of any B vitamins will weaken mitochondria and lead to dysfunction and disease.[357] Evidence continues to grow that mitochondrial dysfunction is the prelude to the development of PD.[358] Folate, a type of B vitamin, is required for the growth and regeneration of mitochondria.[359]

High levels of niacin (Vitamin B3) are found in fish, chicken, turkey, meat, mushrooms, avocados, and peanuts. Niacin is critical for the production of a neuroprotective compound called NAD+ (*nicotinamide adenine dinucleotide*). Recent research suggests that cellular damage caused by misfolded proteins can be reversed by having adequate levels of NAD+.[360]

Folate, vitamins B6, and B12 are the building blocks of the amino acid methionine, which is needed for the vital epigenetic process of methylation. Therefore, B vitamins are needed for healthy gene expression. A low level of Vitamin B6 is associated with a worsening of PD.[361]

B vitamins help to keep levels of the amino acid homocysteine normal. This is of critical importance, as an elevated level of homocysteine has many toxic effects. It contributes to the breakdown of the BBB.[362] It promotes inflammation and may contribute to the development of numerous diseases.[363] High levels of homocysteine contribute to the production of misfolded proteins[364] and weaken dopamine-producing cells.[365] Glutathione (which we will discuss later) is a powerful antioxidant; but high levels of homocysteine lower levels of glutathione.[366]

Folate and Vitamin B6 are found in avocados, beans, spinach, asparagus, broccoli, peppers, cabbage, and other vegetables. Folate is susceptible to high heat; boiling green leafy vegetables reduces the vitamin content by more than 50%. However, steaming does not lower their folate levels.[367] Vitamin B12, found in high levels in meat and fish, lowers levels of homocysteine. A Vitamin B12 deficiency is a risk factor for the development, and worsening of, neurological problems—including PD.[368] Adequate levels of B vitamins work synergistically to lower homocysteine levels[369]—thus helping one's heart, vascular system, and brain.

Foods high in nicotine

As we discuss in an upcoming chapter, it is believed that the protective effect of smoking against PD is because of nicotine.[370] Nicotine raises the levels of detoxifying enzymes in the brain[371] and protects neurotransmitter vesicles.[372] But can we obtain the benefits of nicotine without being exposed to the harmful effects of smoking? Fortunately, nicotine also exists in plants that are related to tobacco: potatoes, tomatoes, eggplants, green peppers,[373] and cauliflower.[374] A recent study found that these foods lower the risk of developing PD.[375]

Glutathione

Many people think that they need to take antioxidants in pill form to help suppress free radicals. In fact, taking antioxidant supplements can be dangerous, as they throw off the natural balance of antioxidants that our bodies have evolved to produce.[376] This is yet another example of the Janus effect, as improper levels of vitamins (such as overdoses) can work against us.[377] Our ancient ancestors did not "pop pills" of 1,000 units of one vitamin and 3,000 units of another vitamin. Our bodies have evolved to benefit from *natural* antioxidants.

One such natural antioxidant is glutathione. **The importance of glutathione cannot be overstated.** The levels of glutathione are 400% higher in the brain than anywhere else in the body.[378] Glutathione also helps to detoxify the brain, suppress neuroinflammation, [379] maintain the integrity of the BBB,[380] and prevent the clumping together of abnormal proteins, such as alpha-synuclein.[381] Moreover, glutathione is involved in the everyday regulation of cellular functions—especially in maintaining the health of mitochondria.[382] Maintaining normal levels of glutathione is proposed to be preventative against neurodegeneration.[383]

Glutathione levels are significantly reduced in the substantia nigra in people with PD—approximately 40% less, as compared to normal people.[384] It is theorized that as glutathione levels drop, iron levels rise, thus triggering higher levels of free radical reactions, neuroinflammation, and death of dopamine-producing cells.[385] Glutathione also plays a major role in protecting another shield—the gut.[386]

Why do glutathione levels drop in Parkinson's Disease? The results of several studies suggest that variations in the genes that produce glutathione and glutathione-related enzymes could be at fault.[387] The effect is most pronounced when people with these variations are exposed to toxins.[388] The LRRK2 gene, associated with the development of PD, may suppress the activity of a glutathione-related enzyme.[389]

It is also possible that exposure to dangerous toxins (such as the pesticide paraquat), simply overwhelm the brain's ability to detoxify, leading to a drastic drop in glutathione levels.[390]

In addition to selenium, glutathione levels are dependent on adequate dietary levels of three amino acids: cysteine, glutamate, and glycine. (Cysteine has another important role in preventing PD. It is also needed for the proper regulation of the transmission and recycling of neurotransmitters, such as dopamine).[391] A diet that is deficient in cysteine, glutamate, and glycine can lead to a deficiency of glutathione in the midbrain *in as little as three days*.[392] Vegans and vegetarians are at risk of glutathione deficiency, due to inadequate cysteine and glycine consumption.[393] In a very interesting study, elderly patients who had low levels of glutathione were given oral supplements of cysteine and glycine for two weeks. Their glutathione levels were restored to that of healthy young people.[394]

In lieu of taking supplements, there are many foods that have adequate amounts of the precursors of glutathione:

> *Cysteine:* The highest levels are found in poultry, pork, and eggs; lower levels are found in garlic, onions, broccoli, beans, peppers, and grains.

> *Glutamate:* The highest levels are found in soy sauce and walnuts; lower levels are found in tomato products, mushrooms, and broccoli.

> *Glycine:* The highest levels are found in pork, whitefish, chicken, turkey, seaweed, and eggs.

It is important to note that glutathione levels are also helped by having adequate exercise and sleep.

Foods that raise levels of uric acid

In various population studies, it was found that people who suffer from gout, a painful arthritic condition, have a lower incidence of PD.[395] Researchers wondered what is it about gout sufferers that predisposes them to attacks of the condition, but at the same time acts in a way to be anti-PD. Medical detectives knew that high levels of uric acid leads to gout; however, metabolites of uric acid, called urates, are in fact potent antioxidants. Urates are neuroprotective against PD. [396] Moreover, urate protects the BBB.[397] Foods that raise uric acid levels include beef, fish, fruits, vegetables, and beer.

Alcoholic and non-alcoholic drinks

We concluded the last paragraph by mentioning beer. In addition to raising levels of uric acid, both alcoholic and non-alcoholic beers contain uridine, which is a component of synaptic membranes.[398] The combination of DHA (found in fish oil) and uridine partially improve dopamine transmission in an animal model of PD.[399] Light to moderate alcohol consumption (1-2 drinks per day) suppresses the mTOR pathway.[400] Drinking one beer a day lowers the risk of developing PD by 5%.[401] Beer raises levels of many cellular antioxidants.[402] If someone prefers wine over beer: there is also a slightly anti-PD effect with the consumption of an occasional glass of wine.[403]

Polyphenols

Polyphenols are beneficial compounds found in plants. A diet rich in polyphenols lowers the risk of developing PD.[404] One substance found in many dozens of plants is kaempferol, which enhances autophagy.[405] Almost all polyphenols cross the BBB and exhibit a wide array of neuropreventative actions:

➢ Anti-inflammation;

➢ Antioxidation;

➢ Chelation of metals;

➢ Protection against neurotoxins;

➢ Reduction of AGEs;

➢ Promotion of new nerve cells (*neurogenesis*);

➢ Protection of the BBB;

➢ Enhancement of natural health-promoting, or *trophic*, factors;

➢ Inhibition of abnormal, misfolded proteins;

➢ Improvement of the gut microbiome;

➢ Gene modulation;
➢ Enhancement of autophagy;

➢ Facilitation of enzymatic reactions;

➢ Provide a food-based source of neurotransmitters.

What follows is an alphabetical listing of some key foods, rich in polyphenols, which are part of the anti-PD diet:

APPLES

The old adage, "an apple a day keeps the doctor away" can be paraphrased to "an apple a day keeps the Parkinson's away."[406] Quercetin, a flavonoid found predominantly in apples (and red onions) prevents mitochondrial damage in the brain.[407] It is also a chelator of iron.[408] Quercetin combined with exercise has a greater benefit for brain health than either exercise or quercetin alone.[409] Quercetin also enhances autophagy [410] and inhibits AGEs.[411]

ASPARAGUS

Asparagus has anti-inflammatory and antioxidant properties. [412] It also can modulate stress pathways.[413] Asparagus is also good for the vascular system, as it is capable of preventing high blood pressure.[414] Extracts of asparagus hold great promise as neuroprotective compounds.[415]

BEETS

Beets are high in several anti-PD compounds:

➤ betaine, which is anti-inflammatory and lowers levels of homocysteine,[416]

➤ luteolin, an antioxidant which is also anti-inflammatory and protective of the BBB;[417]

➤ anthocyanins, which chelate lead and cadmium;[418]

➤ nitrates, which improve cerebral blood flow.[419]

BERRIES

Diets rich in berries, especially blueberries, protect the brain from PD and other neurodegenerative diseases.[420] In addition to protecting dopamine-producing cells, blueberries exert an anti-inflammatory effect.[421] Blueberries significantly enhance dopamine release.[422] Strawberries are high in Vitamin C and fisetin, which is anti-inflammatory, preventative against toxins,[423] and promotes autophagy,[424]

BRASSICA VEGETABLES (BROCCOLI, KALE, BRUSSELS SPROUTS, CABBAGE, CAULIFLOWER, RADISHES, AND TURNIPS)

These vitamin-rich vegetables are highly anti-PD, by supporting multiple shields:

➢ They contain high levels of sulforaphanes, which cross the BBB and maintain levels of aquaporin,[425] which regulates the flow of brain fluids during sleep;

➢ Sulforaphanes also have powerful, beneficial epigenetic properties;[426]

➢ *Brassica* vegetables are also strong inducers of autophagy in protein-misfolding diseases;[427]

➢ They protect against the damage caused by radiation;[428]

➢ They are rich in substances (called *indole-3-carbinol monomers*), which suppress the mTOR pathway;[429]

> ➤ They contain molecules that are essential for the immunity of the intestines.[430]

CHERRIES AND CHERRY JUICE

Cherries (especially tart cherries) and cherry juice contain high levels of melatonin, which is critical in maintaining the normal sleep-wake cycle.[431]

CINNAMON

Cinnamon phenols cross the BBB and have a beneficial effect on astrocytes, a key component of the BBB.[432] It has been shown that extract of cinnamon inhibits the aggregation of alpha-synuclein, making it a substance that is neuroprotective.[433] Levels of the neuroprotective protein DJ-1[434] can be raised by sodium benzoate, a common, safe food additive—which is derived from cinnamon.[435] Both cinnamon and sodium benzoate raise levels of neurotrophic factors in the brain.[436] Cinnamic acid, derived from cinnamon, is a strong inhibitor of AGEs.[437]

COFFEE/CAFFEINE

Caffeinated coffee is a powerful neuroprotective substance. However, it is important to avoid excessive consumption, as caffeine can interfere with sleep. Coffee has the following beneficial properties:

> ➤ it may have an epigenetic effect, modulating the activity of the GRIN2A gene. This gene encodes proteins needed for normal signals within cells;[438]

> ➤ it increases glutathione synthesis, thus raising the level of one of our primary antioxidant shields;[439]

> ➤ it protects the BBB against PD-inducing toxins;[440]

> ➤ it protects the brain against the effects of a high-fat diet;[441]

> ➤ it is anti-inflammatory;[442]

> ➤ it inhibits the mTOR pathway[443] and enhances autophagy;[444]

> ➤ it protects neurotransmitter vesicles against toxins.[445]

CURCUMIN

Curcumin (a derivative of turmeric) is another anti-PD dietary superstar, for the following reasons:

> ➤ it is anti-inflammatory;

> ➤ it inhibits AGEs;[446]

> ➤ it has antioxidant properties and raises levels of glutathione;[447]

> ➤ it has beneficial epigenetic properties;[448]

> ➤ it naturally boosts levels of Heat Shock Proteins;[449]

> ➤ it is a strong inhibitor of alpha-synuclein aggregation;[450]

> ➤ it enhances the activity of lysosomes in order to remove unwanted cellular substances from cells;[451]

➤ it crosses and protects the BBB;[452]

➤ it boosts levels of Brain Derived Neurotrophic Factor (BDNF), thus enhancing the growth and maintenance of new brain connections;[453]

➤ it inhibits the mTOR pathway;[454]

➤ it can chelate iron, copper, lead,[455] and zinc.[456]

GARLIC

Garlic has long been used in folk remedies around the world. Scientists have shown that allicin, a key component of garlic, is a potent antioxidant and has anti-inflammatory properties.[457] Moreover, allicin works synergistically with glutathione.[458] Garlic protects the BBB against the effects of saturated fats.[459] It is also a source of the prebiotic, inulin.

GINGER

There are several beneficial active ingredients derived from ginger: zingerone protects dopamine-producing cells from toxic damage by raising levels of antioxidants;[460] gingerol has potent anti-inflammatory properties;[461] and 6-shogaol, which inhibits the mTOR pathway and enhances autophagy. [462] Ginger is a powerful inhibitor of AGEs.[463]

GRAPES

The skin of red grapes contains a compound called resveratrol. The highest levels of resveratrol are found in red wine.[464] It is well known that the Mediterranean diet is characterized by drinking red wine. The "French paradox," in which it is believed that red wine consumption protects against a high fat diet in France, may be due to resveratrol.[465]

Resveratrol is also found in berries, pistachios and peanuts. There are multiple ways in which resveratrol protects dopamine-producing cells. It prevents excessive inflammation of the glial cells of the BBB, [466] decreases the aggregation of alpha-synuclein,[467] and inhibits the mTOR pathway.[468] It also chelates copper, thereby indirectly lowering iron levels.[469]

In addition to resveratrol, grapes contain other compounds that are anti-inflammatory, antioxidants, and have favorable effects on blood vessels.[470]

GRAPEFRUITS AND ORANGES

Grapefruits and oranges contain high levels of a compound called naringenin (it is also found in the skins of tomatoes). Naringenin has numerous benefits: it penetrates through the BBB, exhibiting anti-inflammatory, antioxidant, and cholesterol-lowering properties. It prevents the loss of dopamine-producing cells when the substantia nigra is exposed to toxins.[471] It also raises levels of neurotrophic factors and suppresses the effects of insulin-like growth factor.[472]

Citrus fruits are high in Vitamin C. Foods rich in Vitamin C inhibit the inflammatory response of the gut triggered by gluten.[473]

Pectin, found in the white inner part of citrus peel, is a strong chelator of metals.[474] Pectin also enhances the growth of the beneficial gut microbe *Faecalibacterium prausnitzii*.[475] This microbe is anti-inflammatory and is linked to a healthy gut.[476]

However, a word of caution before adding grape-fruits (or grapefruit juice) to your diet: more than 85 prescription medications can be dangerously affected by grapefruits and its juice.[477] Check with your doctor or pharmacist to avoid harmful food-drug interactions.

LETTUCE

Lettuce contains many anti-inflammatory and an-tioxidant compounds.[478] It has protective proper-ties against the neurotoxic effects of aluminum.[479]

MUSHROOMS

Mushrooms contain high levels of polyamines, which are powerful antioxidants[480] and induce au-tophagy.[481] Many varieties of mushrooms contains compounds that stimulate nerve growth factors, decrease protein misfolding, and are anti-inflam-matory.[482] Shiitake mushrooms contain trehalose, which helps with clearance of alpha-synuclein.[483]

NUTS, SEEDS, AND GRAINS

Nuts, seeds, and grains are natural sources of Vitamin E, essential fatty acids, melatonin, magnesium, copper, zinc, and folate.

Phytic acid is a compound found in the hulls of nuts, seeds, and grains. It is a potent antioxidant and prevents excessive free radical production caused by iron;[484] it also helps with the detoxification of mercury.[485]

Walnut extract has been shown to protect the BBB against infections; it is also anti-inflammatory.[486] Walnuts decrease the accumulation of misfolded proteins in the brain.[487]

Flax seeds are the best plant-based source of omega-3 fatty acids and are rich in antioxidants.[488] Sesame seeds contain multiple compounds that are anti-inflammatory, antioxidative, and protective for the cells of the BBB.[489] These compounds also chelate iron and lead.[490] In a fascinating study, active ingredients from sesame seeds and oranges reversed the damage induced by a pesticide-induced Parkinson's model in rats.[491]

However, nuts, seeds, and grains should be eaten in small portions, as many have high levels of omega-6 fatty acids.

OLIVE OIL

There are numerous benefits of olive oil. Not only does is it good for the heart and vascular system, but it also has antioxidant properties. It is low in saturated fats and high in beneficial polyphenols. It produces a sense of fullness while eating, thus preventing overeating.[492] Moreover, olive oil prevents neuroinflammatory reactions in the BBB,[493] possibly by inhibiting AGEs.[494] Olive oil promotes normal functioning of the vagus nerve.[495]

The combination of the unsaturated fats of olive oil and nitrites in vegetables create "nitro fatty acids," which lower blood pressure.[496]

Olive oil contains oleocanthal, which has a chemical structure similar to the anti-inflammatory drug ibuprofen. Oleocanthal inhibits the formation of tau, the misfolded protein found in Alzheimer's and in some cases of PD.[497]

Another component of olive oil is oleuropein. It is one of the few known natural substances that can stimulate proteasome activity, thus enhancing the ability of cells to destroy misfolded proteins.[498] Oleuropein also increases levels of protective metallothioneins.[499]

PEPPERS

Peppers (especially red peppers) contain capsaicinoids, which induce autophagy.[500] Pepper, especially when combined with curcumin, protects dopamine-producing cells from the effects of toxins.[501]

PINEAPPLE

Pineapples contain bromelain, which induces autophagy.[502] Bromelain is also anti-inflammatory and is an antioxidant.[503]

ROSEMARY

Rosemary has many anti-PD properties:

➢ It contains betulinic acid, which is one of the few natural substances known to stimulate proteasome activity;[504]

➢ It contains carnosic acid, which protects dopamine-producing cells against the toxic effects of the pesticides dieldrin[505] and rotenone.[506] Carnosic acid is also a powerful antioxidant.[507] It can pass through the BBB and prevent the depletion of glutathione.[508]

➢ It contains the antioxidant rosmarinic acid, which is anti-inflammatory, anti-viral, anti-bacterial,[509] and lowers levels of alpha-synuclein;[510]

The combination of carnosic acid and rosmarinic acid facilitates weight loss by altering levels of gut bacteria.[511]

SOY PRODUCTS

Soybeans contain genistein, an estrogen-like compound. Genistein protects the BBB and dopamine-producing cells from toxins.[512] It is also an antioxidant. [513] However, eating soy products (such as tofu) more than twice a week is associated with the development of dementia in later life.[514]

SPINACH

Spinach has high levels of magnesium, which is needed for brain health. Interestingly, research into the benefits of magnesium for PD was initiated more than fifty years ago. However, the publicity surrounding the drug L-Dopa shifted the efforts of researchers away from studying magnesium.[515]

Magnesium is needed for hundreds of metabolic reactions. It is stored within mitochondria.[516] Magnesium deficiencies are associated with a range of neurodegenerative conditions.[517] People with PD have low concentrations of magnesium in the brain, as compared to people without PD.[518]

In an interesting experiment, magnesium-deficient mice were fed a diet with varying levels of magnesium. The mice were then exposed to MPP+, a neurotoxin that kills dopamine-producing cells. The mice that received low levels of magnesium had partial protection from the toxin: some of their dopamine-producing cells survived.

But those fed a diet high in magnesium had 100% protection from the toxic effects of MPP+. They did not lose any dopamine-producing cells.[519]

There are more reasons why spinach is anti-PD:

➤ Spinach is very high in tryptophan, the precursor for the neurotransmitter serotonin. Maintaining normal levels of serotonin are vital for brain health;[520]

➤ Spinach lowers levels of inflammatory compounds, such as Tumor Necrosis Factor;[521]

➤ The highest levels of folate[522] and betaine,[523] needed to lower homocysteine, are found in spinach;

➤ Magnesium significantly enhances the uptake of dopamine into synaptic vesicles;[524]

➤ Magnesium has been shown to counteract the harmful effects of iron, thus decreasing the aggregation of alpha-synuclein;[525]

➤ Magnesium prevents the depletion of glutathione within brain cells;[526]

➤ Magnesium inhibits some types of calcium channels, thus helping with the critical role of calcium regulation in brain cells;[527]

➤ Spinach binds to toxic metals (arsenic, cadmium, and lead) thus reducing their absorption.[528]

TEAS

Teas have potent neuroprotective capabilities[529] and are associated with a lower risk of PD.[530] There are multiple reasons why teas are highly anti-PD:

➤ Green tea polyphenols inhibit the breakdown of the BBB after brain damage;[531]

➤ Green tea polyphenols inhibit the mTOR pathway;[532]

➤ The active ingredient in green tea is an antioxidant and also chelates iron, thus saving dopamine-producing cells;[533]

➤ Teas have high levels of quinones, which inhibit transglutaminase, the enzyme activated by gluten;[534]

➤ Black tea inhibits the aggregation of alpha-synuclein;[535]

➤ L-theanine (an amino acid) is found predominantly in black tea, with smaller amounts in green tea.[536] It prevents damage caused by several toxins related to PD;[537]

➤ L-theanine protects the brain's blood vessels;[538]

➤ L-theanine raises levels of dopamine and other neurotransmitters;[539]

➤ Green tea,[540] black tea,[541] and oolong tea[542] inhibit the growth of *Streptococcus mutans*;

➤ Another beneficial compound in black tea is theaflavin. It protects neurotransmitter vesicles against free radicals and toxins;[543]

➤ Teas inhibit AGEs.[544]

TOMATOES

Tomatoes have many anti-PD properties:

➤ They have a high nicotine content;

➤ They have naringinen in their skins;

➤ Tomatoes contain lycopene, another potent neuroprotective agent. Higher levels of lycopene are associated with greater survival of dopamine-producing cells.[545] The processing of tomatoes into juice, sauce, paste, and sun-dried tomatoes raises the lycopene concentrations;[546]

➤ Tomatoes, when eaten with fish, inhibit the mTOR pathway;[547]

➤ Tomato paste inhibits AGEs;[548]

➤ Tomatoes are high in lithium. Commonly thought of as a drug solely used for the treatment of psychiatric disorders, recent research has shown the benefit of lithium in neurodegenerative conditions. Lithium enhances autophagy, [549] prevents the death of neurons, functions as an antioxidant, minimizes the aggregation[550] and enhances the clearance of alpha-synuclein[551] while protecting neurotransmitter vesicles. [552] Lithium also stabilizes microtubules, thus protecting the structures of cells, including mitochondria.[553]

➢ Another neuroprotective compound found in tomatoes is lanosterol. [554] Lanosterol protects mitochondria and dopamine-producing cells while increasing autophagy.[555]

YOUR ACTION PLAN

☞ Keep a food diary for a few days, and show it to your doctor. Discuss how your diet can be improved; ask if you need to be seen by a professional Nutritionist or Dietician.

☞ Avoid the Standard American Diet (SAD), which has low levels of fiber and high levels of milk, cheese, salt, unhealthy fats and processed, refined carbohydrates. SAD is a nutrient-depleted diet.

☞ Strive to eat an organic, low-glycemic diet, with a variety of fruits and vegetables, prebiotics and probiotics, extra-virgin olive oil, grains, spices, with small portions of meats, fish, eggs, nuts, and seeds.

Drink several cups of coffee and tea a day. It is okay to have a little wine or beer (alcoholic or non-alcoholic). This diet is low in calories, nutrient-dense, and is anti-PD.

☞ Take nutritional supplements only when medically prescribed (to correct or prevent a specific problem). Remember, vitamins in pill form can throw off the body's balance of natural antioxidants.

☞ Exercise, stress control, sleep, and the avoidance of toxins will help your body to maximize the benefits of good nutrition.

☞ Organic food certification:
http://www.usda.gov/wps/portal/usda/usda-home?navid=ORGANIC_CERTIFICATIO

☞ Understanding mercury levels in fish:
http://www.nrdc.org/health/effects/mercury/guide.asp

☞ Understanding pesticide residues in food:

http://www.ewg.org/foodnews/

5

Exercise

Exercise is a major shield of an anti-PD lifestyle. We will be exploring the numerous benefits of exercise in PD. Unfortunately, once someone develops PD there is a strong likelihood that exercise can be problematic: 70% of people with PD suffer from exercise intolerance due to low levels of neurotransmitters not only in the brain, but also in the heart.[556]

But before we discuss exercise intolerance, let us first mention the dangers of not exercising enough.

THE DANGERS OF SEDENTARY BEHAVIOR

The word "sedentary" comes from the Latin word *sedēre*, to sit. A lifestyle characterized by excessive sitting —being a couch potato—leads to a wide variety of ailments.

Various definitions have been used to characterize "being sedentary:" sitting for more than 5 hours a day; [557] sitting *continuously* for 2 hours or longer, several times a day;[558] walking less than 20 minutes a day;[559] or walking fewer than 5,000 steps per day, as measured with a pedometer.[560] Sedentary behavior leads to an imbalance of the Autonomic Nervous System (ANS)[561] and is associated with an increased risk of hypertension, heart failure,[562] obesity, osteoporosis, constipation, diabetes, [563] cancer,[564] depression, dementia,[565] chronic inflammation,[566] and the worsening of neurodegenerative diseases, such as PD.[567]

How can low levels of exercise worsen PD? There are a variety of mechanisms which probably work in concert. Being sedentary leads to a diminished production of antioxidants[568] and brain repair molecules.[569] The secretion of these compounds is normally dependent upon physical activity.[570] Sedentary behavior is also detrimental for blood flow in the brain, which is regulated by the Blood-Brain Barrier (BBB) and neurotransmitters. Even though the brain makes up only a small percentage of total body weight, it uses approximately 20% of the nutrients and oxygen supplied by the blood.[571] Any impediment to blood circulation is detrimental. Sedentary behavior is a contributor to poor circulation.[572] When circulation is diminished in the brain, it is called *cerebral hypoperfusion*. This is bad for the BBB and is associated with the worsening of brain diseases.[573] A single occurrence of cerebral hypoperfusion, such as during an episode of either high[574] or low blood pressure,[575] leads to further dysfunction of the BBB that may last for weeks.

This is a very real risk for people with PD who have certain types of non-motor problems:

Orthostatic hypotension is one experiences a drop in blood pressure with standing. This can lead to fainting, and to falls;

Post-prandial hypotension is when blood pressure drops after a meal;

Nocturnal hypertension is when blood pressure (which should go down while we sleep) actually spikes up, giving a person high blood pressure while sleeping.

These abnormalities of blood pressure are not rare. It is estimated that up to 60% of people with PD experience such problems[576] and can significantly worsen PD if not medically addressed.

The openings of the BBB (which normally keep out unwanted molecules) widen and remain open, thus allowing toxins to enter the brain.[577] Long-term cerebral hypoperfusion is also unhealthy for the BBB and leads to the death of nerve cells,[578] especially those that produce dopamine.[579] Moreover, cerebral hypoperfusion leads to a buildup of abnormal proteins that normally should be broken down: both of our recycling mechanisms (proteasomes[580] and lysosomes[581]) become dysfunctional. As we have discussed in other chapters, this buildup of abnormal proteins is a hallmark of neurodegeneration.

A poor vascular system, blood pressure problems, high cholesterol, and diabetes are also bad for the blood vessels of the brain,[582] as nutrients cannot reach brain cells. This "starvation" can lead to, and worsen, neurodegeneration.[583] On a genetic level, cerebral hypoperfusion causes detrimental epigenetic changes.[584]

UNDERSTANDING EXERCISE TOLERANCE AND INTOLERANCE

Let us think about the difference between driving two different cars. The first car has tires that are losing air; it is leaking motor oil; and the engine tends to overheat. The second car has absolutely no issues.

The first car can still be driven, but obviously it has its limitations. You can't speed, and you can't take such a car on a long drive.

The second car can be driven for hours at any speed without fear of breaking down or overheating.

70% of people with PD[585] are, unfortunately, like the first car. Just like that problematic car can still drive, these people with PD can still exercise, but at less vigorous intensities. Pushing themselves with exercise raises the risk of developing serious medical issues.

30% of people with PD can exercise at higher intensities and can fully reap the many benefits of exercise. Higher intensity activities can include activities such as brisk walking and biking.

People with PD who are exercise intolerant have significant dysfunctions of the Autonomic Nervous System (ANS). One manifestation of ANS dysfunction has already been discussed: orthostatic hypotension.

Another problem is the inability to perspire normally. They may sweat too little, or too much. As perspiration in a mechanism to regulate body temperature, problems with perspiration can easily lead to overheating. The upshot of this is that the brain will also overheat. Brain cells begin to malfunction when brain temperature rises. In general, people with PD have "hot brains."[586] Exercise-induced overheating will worsen PD.[587]

Another ANS problem that leads to exercise intolerance in PD is called *cardiac denervation*. This means that the heart muscle does not receive the normal supply of norepinephrine (also called noradrenaline; another neurotransmitter that is diminished in PD). [588] With diminished amounts of this neurotransmitter, people with PD fatigue easily. Their hearts simply cannot pump as much blood in response to the demands of movement. Ignoring this limitation has serious risks: abnormal heartbeats, fainting, falling, and even sudden death.[589]

How can we determine who can do only light exercises, and who can do more? Before you start any exercise routine, ask your neurologist to refer you to a cardiologist. In addition to the basic cardiac workup (which includes an electrocardiogram), you may be referred for a test called "MIBG" (the full name is *Cardiac I- metaiodobenzylguanidine scintigraphy*). This test can determine the extent of cardiac denervation, if any. You may also be referred to an autonomic specialist who can determine the extent of perspiration dysfunction. Unfortunately, even a person with mild motor impairment (such as a slight tremor) may already have cardiac issues. There is no correlation between motor and non-motor problems.[590]

Other aspects of PD can also adversely affect one's ability to exercise intensively. If one's muscles are rigid, exercise can cause a severe breakdown of muscle tissue, possibly leading to kidney failure and death. The medical term for this is *rhabdomyolosis*.[591]

The mentality of pushing yourself to your limits, and "no pain, no gain" can be very dangerous. Even a single episode of "overdoing it" can lead to:

> ➢ a significant spike in inflammation;[592]

> ➢ a suppression of the immune system, with an increased risk of infections;[593]

> ➢ musculoskeletal injuries;

> ➢ depletion of key antioxidants;[594]

> ➢ a lowering of magnesium levels, which can last for months;[595]

> ➢ alterations in the ANS;[596]

➢ a weakening of the BBB, especially if exercising in the heat;[597]

➢ an increased uptake of toxins;[598]

➢ degeneration of the locus coeruleus;[599]

➢ sudden death.[600]

Remember, our goal is to minimize neurodegeneration. We don't want to harm ourselves or to "drop dead on the treadmill."

If you are deemed "exercise intolerant," there are still numerous activities that you can enjoy: low intensity exercises such as walking, yoga, Tai Chi, light household work, and stretching. There are many benefits of these types of exercises, and you will be avoiding the PD-related risks of intensive exercise.

A key exercise which is almost always overlooked involves breathing exercises. Enhancing your ability to take deep inhalations and exhalations promotes better oxygen flow. It is important to keep in mind that the main cause of death in PD, pneumonia, involves the lungs.[601] Always try to keep your lungs as healthy as possible, and quickly report any difficulties in breathing to your doctor.

EXERCISE: BENEFITS FROM THE VIEWPOINT OF EPIGENETICS

Exercise has profound effects on the "turning on" or the "turning off" of genes. This is a dynamic, lifelong process.[602] The most commonly studied epigenetic process is *methylation*. Abnormalities in methylation are common in PD; in particular, epigenetic regulation of alpha-synuclein is abnormal.[603] Exercise is a powerful regulator of methylation. The epigenetic benefits can begin with the first workout.[604] Regular practitioners of Tai Chi have improved methylation.[605]

EXERCISE INCREASES LEVELS OF ANTIOXIDANTS

Neurodegenerative diseases are characterized by low levels of brain antioxidants;[606] it is possible that low levels of antioxidants contribute to the onset of PD. Diminished levels of brain antioxidants are dangerous to the supporting structures that form a framework within cells. Any malfunction of these supports can cause abnormal proteins—which should be transported out, earmarked for disposal—to be trapped inside brain cells.[607] Unfortunately, the cellular supports of dopamine-producing cells appear to be especially vulnerable.[608] It is therefore absolutely critical to maintain high levels of antioxidants. This can be accomplished through sleep, diet, and regular exercise.

EXERCISE INCREASES LEVELS OF NEUROTROPHIC FACTORS

Our bodies produce beneficial molecules called neurotrophic factors. They are needed for the growth, functioning, and repair of nerve cells throughout the nervous system. Dr. Carl Cotman, an expert in brain aging, calls them "brain fertilizer."[609] Low levels of these factors are found in PD and other neurodegenerative diseases.[610]

Many neurotrophic factors have been identified and researched. Increased levels of neurotrophic factors are also associated with improved mood, memory, sleep, and reversal of obesity. Fortunately, the levels of these critically important molecules can be augmented through regular exercise:[611]

➤ GDNF (Glial cell line-derived neurotrophic factor) and BDNF (Brain-derived neurotrophic factor) [612] protect dopamine-producing neurons from toxins.[613] GDNF can also strengthen previously damaged cells;[614]

➤ VEGF (Vascular endothelial growth factor) and IGF-1 (Insulin-like growth factor-1) are needed for the growth of new blood vessels and new nerve connections in the brain and nervous system.[615] IGF-1 also protects against toxins;[616]

➤ CDNF (Cerebral Dopamine Neurotrophic Factor), which specifically protects dopamine-producing cells from toxins, with an effect far greater than that of other neurotrophic factors;[617]

➤ VIP (Vasoactive Intestinal Peptide): Triggered by exercise,[618] VIP has a dramatic effect on sleep. VIP induces REM sleep and regulates circadian rhythms.[619] It also protects against the loss of dopamine producing cells, raises levels of the neurotransmitters GABA and prevents neuroinflammation. [620] VIP induces the release of ADNP (Activity Dependent Neuroprotective Protein)[621] which protects mitochondria in PD.[622]

EXERCISE HELPS THE GUT

There are several ways in which exercise is beneficial for the gut. Exercise decreases constipation.[623] In terms of gut bacteria, exercise decreases the effects of toxins[624] and promotes the growth of a diverse set of organisms.[625] Abnormal levels of gut organisms, associated with obesity and hypertension, can be altered through exercise.[626]

EXERCISE INTEGRATES SENSORY MESSAGES AND MODULATES THE RELEASE OF NEUROTRANSMITTERS

Although movement is usually thought of as a series of muscle contractions, it is also a series of sensations. To illustrate: let's say you are playing tennis. You *hear* and *see* the ball being hit to you; you run to the side, *feeling* the impact of your feet on the court; you extend your elbow while gripping the racket, and quickly contact other muscles to hit the ball in return. While this is happening, the *vestibular system* (within your inner ears) makes sure that you keep your balance. It only takes milliseconds for vision, sound, muscle tension and vestibular sensations to be blended together in the brain and for you to make the appropriate movement.

In a normal person, the striatum[627] (a portion of the basal ganglia)[628] integrates sensory signals and responds by releasing dopamine, thus facilitating the appropriate muscle response. Regular exercise training increases the efficiency of the striatum.[629] However, there is deterioration of the basal ganglia in PD. The result: sensory integration, and the dopamine response, is diminished.[630] Deep Brain Stimulation helps patients with PD to move better because the procedure improves dopamine release from the striatum.[631]

Exercise raises levels of other neurotransmitters besides dopamine. Depression is one of the problems of PD; it is believed to be caused by abnormal levels of serotonin and other neurotransmitters.[632] Exercise has the potential to restore imbalances of neurotransmitters in depression.[633]

BUILDING UP COGNITIVE RESERVE: ANOTHER TYPE OF EXERCISE

Although dementia is generally associated with Alzheimer's Disease, some types of PD also have an element of dementia. Deterioration of the locus coeruleus is linked to poor mental status in these diseases.[634] Higher levels of education are associated with lower levels of dementia in PD.[635] Other activities that are beneficial include reading, playing a musical instrument, learning a second language, engaging in problem solving and being socially engaged. All of these activities build up "cognitive reserve:" the ability to avoid or minimize dementia despite having a neurodegenerative disease.[636] Similar to the actions of physical exercise, mental exercise also triggers increased activation of neurotransmitters,[637] neurogenesis, BDNF, and brain activity.[638] "Brain exercises" may therefore reduce the risk of dementia.

YOUR ACTION PLAN

☞   Before starting an exercise program, go to your doctor. It is important to discuss any non-motor problems (such as low blood pressure upon standing). It is also prudent to ask for a referral to an autonomic specialist for a detailed analysis of your blood pressure, heart response, and ability to perspire.

☞   If you need professional guidance on managing a fitness program, ask your doctor for referrals to a physical therapist and other members of the rehabiliatation team (such as an occupational therapist and a speech therapist). A physical therapist can address any issues that you might have with your posture, your balance, your flexibility, your strength, and your ability to walk. Remember, no two patients with PD are exactly alike. Physical therapists specialize in developing individualized care based not only their initial evaluations, but also on your progress as you begin to show improvements;

☞   Avoid: over-exercising and dehydration;

☞   Exercise in a cool, well-ventilated environment.

6

Sleep and the Light-Dark Cycle

We spend one-third of our lives asleep. Sleep is a physiological need. Sleeping between 6 and 8 hours per night is related to good health (especially brain health).[639] Even one night of partial sleep deprivation is enough to alter body chemistry. For example, having only a few hours of sleep can cause a 24-hour loss of insulin sensitivity by up to 25%.[640]

Virtually all people with PD will eventually suffer from poor sleep. [641] Excessive sleepiness during the day strongly suggests that one's nighttime sleep is not restorative.

Besides PD, other sleep-related factors must also be evaluated. For example, is it a urinary problem (such as an enlarged prostate in men) that causes frequent bathroom trips at night, thus fragmenting sleep? Is the bed uncomfortable? Is the bedroom too warm? Does the spouse snore? Does the person stay up half the night watching television? Does arthritic pain make it hard to find a comfortable position? Does the person drink caffeinated drinks late at night, thus causing unneeded stimulation to the brain?

Improving the quality of sleep is critically important in managing PD. It is hypothesized that early recognition and treatment of sleep disorders can alleviate the early non-motor aspects of PD, thus preventing further disability.[642]

If your doctor feels that you need an overnight sleep study in a sleep laboratory, the following sleep problems can be detected:

Insomnia: People with insomnia can fall asleep, but they cannot stay asleep. Insomnia may be successfully treated with medications, or with BLT: Bright Light Therapy.

In several studies, people with insomnia (including some with PD) were exposed to bright lights that were at least 1,000 lux up to 7,500 lux ("lux" is a measure of brightness), for 30-90 minutes either in the morning or before they went to sleep. The majority of the people felt that their insomnia was significantly improved.[643]

Nocturnal hypertension: Blood pressure is supposed to go down at night, but for some people with PD, their blood pressure rises at night. This is a very dangerous non-motor problem, as it worsens PD during sleep, as well as potentially damaging the heart.[644] Once detected, it can be treated with blood pressure medications to be taken before bedtime.

Restless leg syndrome: This is not uncommon in PD. It is a sleep-related movement disorder in which the person has an uncontrollable urge to move their legs. Although it is sometimes treated with PD medications, one study showed that supplementation with magnesium at nighttime significantly improved total sleep time, with fewer arousals due to restless legs.[645]

Sleep apnea: The stoppage of breathing during sleep is another very dangerous condition, as it can lead to drops in oxygen and spikes in blood pressure. Both of these are bad for the brain and the heart. Fortunately, it can successfully be treated with a Continuous Pressure Airway Pressure (CPAP) device.

REM Sleep Behavior Disorder: Normal sleep is characterized by various stages of brain activity. Each stage has specific health-enhancing benefits. Sleep is broadly categorized into Rapid Eye Movement (REM) and Non-REM (NREM) sleep:

REM sleep: This is when we dream, and our eyes quickly twitch back and forth. However, the muscles of our body are turned off. REM sleep is associated with energy restoration and the support of daytime activities. It is during REM sleep that the growth of new nerve connections take place, neurotransmitter levels are restored, and the cells of the BBB become strengthened.[646]

NREM sleep: Broken down into stages 1-4; the later stages are associated with a decrease in the production of the stress hormone, cortisol; the cooling of the brain and body; the lowering of blood pressure; the release of hormones, and the overall repair of the body.

As we just described, during normal sleep, people do not move while they dream. But people who suffer from REM Sleep Behavior Disorder do not stay still. Their movements tend to follow the content of their dreams. The movements may be as simple as jerking limbs or they may involve screaming, thrashing about, kicking, or punching. It is not uncommon for these people to injure themselves or their bed partners. People with REM Sleep Behavior Disorder, and their bed partners, must be aware of the safety of their sleeping environment.

REM Sleep Behavior Disorder is not easy to treat. Various medications have been tried, with limited success.

THE LIGHT-DARK CYCLE AND CIRCADIAN RHYTHMS

Humans, like all other life forms, evolved on earth over the course of millions of years. Our bodies adapted to the daily cycle of approximately 12 hours of light from the sun and approximately 12 hours of darkness.

When light hits the retinas of our eyes, an amazing chain of biological events is initiated. Specialized nerve endings—called photoreceptors — become stimulated. They send a nerve impulse to an area deep within the brain. The target of this impulse is a group of cells in the hypothalamus. The technical term for this group of cells is the *suprachiasmatic nucleus*. It can be thought of as a natural pacemaker, or as a biological clock. The suprachiasmatic nucleus controls the natural rhythms of the body, known as circadian rhythms (circadian means "about a day").

The suprachiasmatic nucleus is usually resistant to a wide range of toxins.[647] It has to be, as it does not have the protection of the Blood-Brain Barrier (BBB). However, some toxins can cause subtle changes to the mitochondria of the suprachiasmatic nucleus. This leads to circadian disruption, sleep disturbances, and may worsen neurodegeneration.[648]

The suprachiasmatic nucleus also sends signals to the pineal gland. This tiny structure—about the size of a grain of rice—produces melatonin. We will discuss melatonin later; let's first discuss the importance of circadian rhythms.

Circadian rhythms are critical for health. Regular patterns of gene activation, hunger, digestion, hormone release, immune response, neurotransmitter release, urine flow, body temperature fluctuation, cellular repair, response to medications, and sleep are just some of our bodily functions that undergo patterns during a 24-hour period. Disruption of this regular cycle usually results in disease. It has been shown in insects that disrupting circadian rhythms not only speeds up aging but it can worsen neurodegeneration.[649]

The cellular structures that degrade and recycle abnormal, misfolded proteins include the proteasome and the lysosome. They follow a circadian rhythm. Poor sleep patterns disrupt the functioning of proteasomes[650] and lysosomes,[651] thus increasing the risk of neurodegeneration.

Another shield that is regulated by circadian rhythms is the gut. When sleep patterns are poor, alterations in gut bacteria occur, thus contributing to inflammation, obesity, and a leaky gut.[652]

The circadian rhythm is regulated by specific sleep-related genes; more than 100 have been identified.[653] These genes activate the 24-hour regulation of biological functions in the brain and the rest of the body. When one's sleep cycle is altered, more than 1,300 genes fail to function normally;[654] but when one becomes sleep deprived, the effect is much more devastating. It has been estimated that more than 4,000 genes are affected. Many of these are involved in the production of proteins, antioxidants, cellular protectants, and the storage of neurotransmitters.[655]

Insufficient sleep also alters the genes for immune function, response to stress, triglyceride metabolism, hormonal responses, and epigenetic functions.[656] When one of the epigenetic processes (such as methylation) fails, our sleep can suffer even more. Decreased methylation of sleep genes is found in people with PD.[657] Epigenetic processes involving microRNAs also become dysfunctional, and cause abnormalities in the production of a key antioxidant, glutathione. [658] As dopamine levels begin to drop, the genes regulating the circadian clock begin to fail.[659] In a vicious cycle, the loss of sleep then causes additional alterations of gene expression and further disruption of the circadian clock.[660] Without adequate sleep, our cellular shields do not function properly.[661]

Studies have been done in insects and animals to test what happens when sleep genes are "knocked out," or deactivated: memory becomes impaired; movements become slow; and inflammation of the BBB is initiated. In short, when sleep genes fail, brain activity worsens.[662]

SUNLIGHT AND VITAMIN D

It is important to note that there are other important biological functions of properly-timed light, especially sunlight. In addition to synchronizing the biological clock, our bodies use sunlight to produce Vitamin D. High levels of Vitamin D lower the risk of developing PD by 67%.[663] Vitamin D is required for the proper functioning of approximately 3,000 genes.[664] Some of these genes are absolutely critical for brain health, such as the one that activates the production of the neurotransmitter serotonin.[665] The highest concentration of Vitamin D receptors are found in the midbrain—where dopamine is produced.[666] Unfortunately, it is estimated that more than half of the world's population is at risk of Vitamin D deficiency.[667]

There are many other anti-PD benefits of having healthy levels of Vitamin D:

➢ it induces autophagy;[668]

➢ it is beneficial for the gut and immune system;[669]

➢ it raises levels of the brain antioxidant, glutathione;[670]

➢ it reduces pain;[671]

➢ it aids with clearance of toxins and lowering of homocysteine;[672]

➢ it is a regulator of iron levels;[673]

➢ it triggers the production of neurotrophin, nerve growth factor, and glial cell-line derived neurotrophic factor (GDNF);[674]

> ➢ it regulates calcium levels in cells.[675] This is critically important, as abnormalities in calcium flow makes dopamine-producing cells more vulnerable to the effects of toxins.[676]

Moreover, sunlight activates nitrate and nitrate-related molecules (obtained from a vegetable-rich diet), which are stored in the skin.[677] Nitrates and nitrites are used to produce nitric oxide, which functions as an immune booster,[678] a neurotransmitter,[679] and a vasodilator.[680] Some studies have found that nitric oxide levels are reduced in PD, Alzheimer's, and other neurological diseases.[681] Nitric oxide may protect against neurodegeneration.[682]

Therefore, sun exposure is beneficial for a variety of reasons. The key is to avoid sunburn. It is recommended to spend time outdoors during the summer and to take Vitamin D supplements (only with the approval of your doctor) during the other seasons.[683]

MELATONIN

Melatonin, a hormone, may rank as the most amazing naturally-produced chemical. Melatonin is suppressed by light; it is secreted during darkness. This pattern is critical for health.

Melatonin rapidly passes through the BBB and is stored throughout the nervous system.[684] Melatonin levels decline with aging. This may explain why the most common neurodegenerative diseases, Alzheimer's and PD, occur primarily in the elderly.[685]

Dr. Russel J. Reiter, a giant in the field of melatonin research, has aptly called melatonin "a multitasking molecule." [686] There are numerous anti-PD benefits of melatonin:

➢ it promotes sleep;

➢ it protects against a leaky gut;[687]

➢ it stimulates beneficial epigenetic processes;[688]

➢ it is an extremely potent antioxidant. Moreover, it also augments levels of glutathione (discussed in the Diet chapter). Therefore, a good night's sleep raises levels of our two most powerful natural antioxidants; [689]

➢ it strengthens the immune system;

➢ it benefits the cardiovascular system;

➢ it prevents mitochondria damage, which is a significant contributor to the aging process;[690]

➢ it helps neurogenesis;[691]

➢ it protects the BBB[692] and substantia nigra from the damaging effects of a wide range of chemicals.[693] Melatonin has been shown to be somewhat protective against exposures to pesticides,[694] fungicides, and other toxins.[695] It has been proposed that some toxins have the potential to trigger PD by interfering with nightly melatonin secretion patterns;[696]

➢ it minimizes damage to the brain caused by radiation;[697]

➢ it regulates obesity;[698]

➢ it blocks the formation of alpha-synuclein, the misfolded protein associated with PD;[699]

➢ it protects neurotransmitter vesicles from toxins;[700]

> ➢ it lessens the severity of many mood disorders.[701]

HOW SLEEP PREVENTS BRAIN DEGENERATION: THE ACTIVATION OF THE GLYMPHATIC SYSTEM

Dr. Maiken Nedergaard and her team of researchers of the University of Rochester Medical Center made a discovery that has a profound understanding of the science of sleep. They found that during sleep there is a 60% increase in the space between the membranes of the brain. This increase in space allows brain fluids to increase their flow. This "rinse cycle" allows the brain to rid itself of abnormal proteins that accumulate during the day. The flow of the fluids is along previously unidentified channels, which Dr. Nedergaard has dubbed "the glymphatic system." [702]

The BBB is an important part of the story. A key protein messenger involved in the glymphatic system is aquaporin 4, or AQP4. The job of AQP4 is to facilitate the flow of fluids. It is produced in the BBB.[703]

Although Dr. Nedergaard's research focused on the clearance of beta-amyloid (the abnormal protein associated with Alzheimer's Disease), the same holds true for the clearance of alpha-synuclein, the abnormal protein associated with PD. It has been shown by other researchers that low levels of AQP4 lower the defenses of the brain to PD-producing agents.[704] Levels of AQP4 are also associated with neuroinflammation[705] and the severity of PD.[706] Therefore, a good night's sleep is restorative and neuropreventative is because toxins and abnormal proteins are removed via the glymphatic system.

In a related study, it was found that loss of sleep for just one night causes a sharp rise in blood levels of two BBB-related compounds. These chemicals, S-110B and the enzyme NSE, are usually associated with damage to neurons,[707] such as the neurodegeneration caused by a traumatic brain injury. A loss of sleep for one night does not cause the same damage to the BBB as a blow to the head, but it is bad for the brain.[708]

THE DANGER OF EXCESSIVE LIGHT EXPOSURE: CHRONODISRUPTION

We can turn on televisions, computers, or hand-held devices at any time. Although this is an example of mankind's technological prowess, it is also a curse of our modern society. Light at night has two potentially devastating effects: our circadian rhythms can become altered, and our melatonin levels can be suppressed. As a result, there could be alterations in biological patterns as well as an increase in free-radicals, both of which are implicated in neurodegeneration, cancer, and other diseases.[709]

ADDITIONAL LIFESTYLE FACTORS THAT REGULATE SLEEP

Diet

A Mediterranean diet has numerous health-enhancing benefits. We can add improved sleep to the list. In particular, the optimal ratio of essential fatty acids appears to play a key role in sleep.[710] Extra virgin olive oil has high levels of melatonin,[711] and it may be one reason why people who adhere to a Mediterranean diet have such a low incidence of neurodegenerative disorders.[712] Other components of a Mediterranean diet are also rich in melatonin: it is present in fruits, vegetables, nuts, grains, wine, herbs and spices.[713]

Spinach and beets are high in nitrates and nitrites, needed for the production of nitric oxide.

Broccoli is high in aquaporin 4, needed for optimization of the glymphatic system.

Exercise

Although exercise is not as powerful as light in terms of synchronizing circadian rhythms, it can have a significant effect.[714] Exercising, especially at a consistent time of the day (such as taking a walk at lunchtime), may also enhance melatonin release.[715]

Another chemical produced by the body during exercise is VIP (Vasoactive Intestinal Polypeptide). VIP helps to regulate sleep. It accomplishes this by synchronizing the circadian rhythms.[716]

Obesity

Fat cells are not inert packing material. Each fat cell is biologically active. In terms of sleep, fat cells can alter metabolic circadian rhythms.[717] Obesity has the potential to impair sleep, and poor sleep has the potential to cause weight gain. It is thought that poor sleep leads to increased cravings for high-carbohydrate and high-fat foods.[718] Moreover, as body weight increases, so does the risk of developing obstructive sleep apnea.[719] As with many regulators of sleep, the connections are multifaceted: hormones that control hunger and a sense of fullness after eating are also part of the sleep-wake cycle.[720]

Stress

There is an association between stress, Brain-Derived Neurotrophic Factor (BDNF), and insomnia. Moreover, the connection is multidirectional. Insomnia leads to increased stress, and therefore less BDNF, which worsens insomnia. Increased stress during the day can reduce levels of BDNF, leading to poor sleep.[721] It is important to break this vicious cycle, as it is detrimental to the brain.

YOUR ACTION PLAN

 If you feel tired during the day, you might have a PD-related sleep disorder. Talk to you doctor about your problem. You may be referred for an overnight sleep study, preferably at a sleep laboratory that has been accredited by the American Academy of Sleep Medicine:

http://www.sleepeducation.com/find-a-center

☞   In order to maintain a healthy circadian rhythm, avoid darkness during the day and avoid light at night. Remember, nighttime is for sleeping.

☞   Inexpensive devices can be used to block out light and noise at night: eyeshades and earplugs have been associated with improved REM sleep and increased melatonin release.[722]

☞   Avoid the usage of electronic devices at night; keep them away from your bed (even if you are simply charging them).

☞   Remember the other lifestyle factors: a healthy diet, regular exercise, avoidance of obesity, and stress reduction. Each shield plays a role in the improvement of sleep.

☞   Sun exposure during the day is important; avoid sunburns.

☞   Ask your doctor to check your Vitamin D level.

7

Stress Management

Any stressful incident, or a "stressor," sounds an alarm: it triggers a cascade of events in the nervous system. Stressors can be actual events, or they may be anticipated. Some events are short-lived, while other events can be chronic.

Imagine that you are walking down the street. Suddenly a car swerves out of control and jumps the sidewalk. Your brain detects the stressor—an out of control car— and your brain releases several hormones; they in turn trigger neurotransmitters. The hormones and neurotransmitters instantly allow a dramatic increase in blood flow to your heart and legs, allowing you to run out of the way. Just as our cavemen ancestors ran away from angry lions, we have the same survival mechanism that allows us to escape harm from a sudden, short-term stressor. This is referred to as *acute* stress, or the "fight or flight" response.

The effect of acute stress on the Blood-Brain-Barrier (BBB) is dramatic. It has been demonstrated in rats (whose BBB is similar to ours) that even brief stressors (lasting between 4[723] and 30 minutes[724]) cause an alteration of the protective function of the BBB. The negative consequences of this acute stress last for hours. This suggests that having a "bad day"—for example, triggered by a heated argument with family member or co-worker—can temporarily cause openings in your BBB.

Acute stress also causes significant changes in dopamine release in various regions of the brain, with increases ranging from 25% to 95% above baseline.[725] It is possible that repeated stress leads to a depletion of dopamine.

CHRONIC STRESS, THE BRAIN, AND PD

Repeated, long-term stress is referred to as *chronic* stress. It is usually characterized by a sense that you have no control over a situation. Just as physical stress to the brain (a Traumatic Brain Injury) is linked to PD, chronic *emotional* stress is also linked to PD.

Chronic stress has a negative effect on our shields:

➤ Chronic stress alters the normal protective function of the BBB;[726]

➤ Stress hormones and neurotransmitters impair blood flow to dopamine-producing cells, thus accelerating dopamine loss;[727]

➤ The locus coeruleus, the key regulator of norepinephrine release, demonstrates significant problems with prolonged stress.[728] Loss of these cells, due to stress, can be manifested as depression[729]—one of the preclinical problems of PD. It theorized that abnormalities of the locus coeruleus "sets the stage" for degeneration of dopamine-producing cells;[730]

➤ Chronic stress triggers genetic changes, such as the genes that are involved with the flow of calcium into cells. It has been proposed that stress-induced dysfunction of these genes contribute to Alzheimer's[731] and PD;[732]

➤ Chronic stress lowers levels of Brain-Derived Neurotrophic Factor (BDNF);[733]

➤ The cascade of hormones, inflammatory compounds, and other chemical messengers produced by chronic stress can trigger, and worsen, neuroinflammation;[734]

➤ Chronic stress impairs the growth of new brain cells. In particular, one area of the brain that is worsened by stress is the hippocampus. As the hippocampus malfunctions, the symptoms of depression can appear. This, in turn, worsens coping mechanisms, thus creating a vicious cycle of decreased growth of new brain cells and depression.[735] Stress, if combined with depression, poor sleep, high levels of inflammation, and sedentary behavior significantly impairs the growth of new brain cells.[736]

➤ Whereas acute stress temporarily boosts immunity, chronic stress lowers immunity;[737]

➤ Chronic stress is extremely bad for the gut. Blood flow decreases; digestion becomes slowed; the unhealthy organisms of the microbiome increase; the intestines become more open to toxins; and the Autonomic Nervous System suffers;[738]

STRESS MANAGEMENT: RELAXATION

"Relaxation" is a state in which deep rest leads to the reduction of stress and enhances wellness. In short, it is the opposite of the "fight or flight" response. The benefits of the relaxation extend way beyond our minds: a recent study found that people who regularly practice relaxation techniques enjoy the triggering of genes that are involved in a healthy immune system, insulin secretion, and energy use. Short-term practice initiates these effects and long-term practice further increases the benefits. [739] Meditation also reduces the thinning of several brain regions which normally occur with aging.[740] It also improves the responsiveness of the vagus nerve [741] and enhances dopamine production.

There is a case of a man who was diagnosed with PD. The diagnosis was verified through a DaT scan. A religious man, he had practiced meditation for many years. Meditating did not prevent his onset of PD, but he continued with his daily, 30 minutes of meditation. After 16 years of meditating, he felt that his PD was gone. He discussed this with his neurologist, who ordered a repeat DaT scan.

Amazingly, his new scan was perfectly normal, with no signs of PD. It is very possible that his daily meditation enhanced recovery of his brain. However, his other lifestyle factors were not studied, so we cannot be absolutely certain that it was only meditation that was helpful.[742]

The bottom line is that meditation, which is known to enhance dopamine production, *may* help someone with PD. And there are no harmful side effects!

Other types of relaxation techniques:

> ➤ Deep breathing;

> ➤ Hypnosis;

> ➤ Biofeedback;

> ➤ Prayer;

> ➤ Exercise (such as gentle, non-competitive exercises, like Tai Chi or yoga);

> ➤ Psychotherapy. The value of emotionally supportive healthcare providers is of the utmost importance in order to ease the stress of PD, Specialists in the field of psychology can

provide vital, one-on-one, personalized care to hopefully minimize stress, anxiety, depression, and relaxation for people with PD. They can also teach one how to meditate.

YOUR ACTION PLAN

☞ Take time each day to practice a stress management technique. The benefits can be achieved with as little as 15 minutes a day of relaxation (but as per the previously discussed case, 30 minutes may be better);[743]

☞ Keep the other shields healthy: diet, exercise, sleep.

☞ Do not keep your feelings of stress, depression, or anxiety bottled up. Share them with a friend, loved one, or a psychologist.

☞ Avoid social isolation.

☞ Healthy Ways to Cope with Stress:

http://www.cdc.gov/violenceprevention/pub/coping_with_stress_tips.html

8

Avoidance of Toxins

In 2005, eleven Canadians agreed to have their blood tested by Environmental Defence, a nonprofit environmental group.

Each person was tested for 88 contaminants, including pesticides, flame retardants, stain cleaners, and heavy metals. These substances are linked to a wide range of illnesses including neurodegenerative diseases, cancer, reproductive disorders, and respiratory conditions.

The people who were tested came from various parts of Canada.

The results: on average, each person tested positive for 44 chemicals.

What does this tell us? That probably everyone on the planet—not just Canadians—is exposed to a host of harmful chemicals. Each and every one of us becomes a reservoir of our polluted, toxic environment.

Let's discuss the different categories of harmful substances: those found in air pollution; bug and weed killers; metals; solvents; and PCBs. We will also discuss the dangers of smoking, drug use, and the toxic effects of radiation.

AIR POLLUTION

The air quality in Mexico City has been steadily improving for the past several years. This is a result of concerted actions by environmental groups and government policies. But just a few years ago the situation was much different. Not only was the air in Mexico City bad; it was dangerous to breath.

The effects of air pollution were extensively studied by Dr. Lilian Calderón-Garcidueñas. She and her team of researchers studied the effects of air pollution on children and adults who spent considerable time in the streets of Mexico City.

The researchers found that inhaling the gases and particles found in polluted air creates a cascade of harmful events in the human body. The first insult is to the cells of the nasal passages. When these cells are exposed, their protective function becomes weakened. Moreover, toxins pass into and weaken the defenses of the Blood-Brain Barrier (BBB).[744] The weakening of the BBB allows the particulate matter to trigger brain inflammation. All of the subjects tested by Dr. Calderón-Garcidueñas's team showed the same pattern of respiratory and brain dysfunction. In older adults, these changes may be blamed on aging. But the researchers found that even children exhibited brain changes identical with early Parkinson's and Alzheimers.[745] In a follow-up study, Calderón-Garcidueñas found that children exposed to pollution had immune responses to formaldehyde, benzene, bisphenol A, nickel, and cadmium.[746] By the time these children age into their 30s, their brains exhibit neuroinflammation with an accumulation of manganese, cobalt, and selenium.[747]

Across the world in Belgium, another team of researchers studied the effects of exercising when air pollution levels are high. Maintaining a high aerobic fitness level improves brain function by decreasing brain inflammation and enhancing the release of naturally protective brain chemicals. Aerobically fit people perform well not only on tests that measure their physical fitness, but also on tests of their cognitive (thinking and reasoning) skills. But the researchers found that people who exercise in polluted environments—such as those who jog alongside a busy highway—lose some of the beneficial effects of exercise. Their physical fitness may improve, but their cognitive fitness does not.[748]

The exhaust from diesel vehicles is especially dangerous. An American research team determined that chronic exposure to diesel fumes triggers inflammation and degeneration in the substantia nigra. [749]

Air pollution triggers deleterious reactions in the body, far beyond the effects of the nasal passages, lungs, and brain. It has been demonstrated that air pollution has the potential to alter normal gene expression in various organs, cause inflammatory responses, and to initiate hormonal changes similar to those produced in stressful situations.[750] Particulate matter can trigger a leaky gut, which adds to inflammation.[751] Autonomic responses (such as the heart's response to exercise) are diminished when air pollution levels are high.[752]

PESTICIDES, FUNGICIDES, HERBICIDES

In July 1982, a 42 year - old man arrived at Santa Clara Valley Medical Center in San Jose, California. What was unusual about this man was that he was frozen in a grotesque posture—not unlike someone with end-stage PD. In a fascinating medical detective story, the hospital's Chief Neurologist, Dr. J. William Langston, determined that the patient (and six other local patients) had tried a new type of synthetic heroin.

Researchers ultimately discovered that the heroin was not truly heroin. What had accidentally been created was a known, toxic substance called MPTP. Thus, began a new chapter in the understanding of PD: the disease could be directly triggered by exposure to a harmful chemical.[753]

MPTP exerts its toxic effect on people by disrupting the mitochondria of dopamine-producing cells. But there is a well-known class of chemicals that also exert their effect on living species by disrupting the inner workings of mitochondria: pesticides. In fact, a commonly used pesticide, paraquat, is very similar in chemical structure to MPTP.[754] Paraquat causes an increase in levels of alpha-synuclein,[755] probably by inhibiting the proteasome system[756] (which normally degrades abnormal proteins).

A wide range of pesticides cause genetic and/or epigenetic damage.[757] There is a growing body of evidence that in addition to paraquat, exposures to other pesticides (as well as fungus killers, or fungicides, and weed-killers, or herbicides) may significantly raise the risk of developing PD: maneb/mancozeb,[758] rotenone,[759] Agent Orange,[760] and many others.[761] Chronic rotenone exposure disrupts the cellular defense systems which degrade abnormal proteins; it alters DJ-1, a protective protein; and it triggers high levels of alpha-synuclein.[762] Rotenone, although toxic, may actually be considered "organic," as it is derived from the roots of tropical plants. However, there is a growing awareness of the dangers of including this substance in organic gardening.[763]

But what about the rest of us, who are not farmers? Are we at risk of developing PD due to pesticide exposures? Consider this:

> Although many dangerous pesticides have been banned in America for private use, the residues of some chemicals continue to exist in the environment. For example, benomyl, a banned pesticide,

lingers in the soil and has the potential to damage dopamine-producing cells;[764]

➤ Even amateur gardeners have a slightly elevated risk of PD, due to use of bug and weed-killers;[765]

➤ Living in a house that had been fumigated increases the risk of PD;[766]

➤ It is possible for the runoff of pesticides to get into private wells. In some communities, well-water consumption increases the risk of PD;[767]

➤ For people with genetic vulnerabilities, even low levels of exposures to pesticides can trigger a cascade of reactions that lead to epigenetic dysfunction, and ultimately, the death of dopamine-producing cells;[768]

➤ Asymptomatic agricultural workers—those who have been exposed to pesticides but did not develop PD—have brain damage similar to PD, but to a lesser extent.[769]

METALS

We need to consume small trace amounts of certain metals for optimal health. For this reason, they are called essential metals. Iron, zinc, manganese, copper and a few others fit into this category. Copper and zinc are needed by the body to produce a potent antioxidant, Copper-Zinc Superoxide Dismutase, or CuZnSOD for short. But inadequate or excessive levels of essential metals can result in disease. The body has very intricate processes to regulate some of these metals, such as copper and iron.[770] When copper regulation fails, iron levels rise and may contribute to the onset of PD.[771] The complex role of copper and PD requires further research.[772]

High levels of metals can not only be toxic to the brain, but they also throw off the chemistry of the gut—thus having the potential of triggering a wide range of diseases.[773] Moreover, some metals (such as aluminum and mercury) are not part of normal human biology and can have toxic effects, even at minute levels. Dr. Vladimir Uversky and Dr. Anthony Fink are among the world's foremost experts on the triggers of alpha-synuclein. They have found that metals trigger the formation of alpha-synuclein.[774] They have also found that metals, combined with pesticides, work synergistically to accelerate the formation of alpha-synuclein.[775] Metals can interrupt the normal "symphony" of events that take place at nerve synapses: the production of neurotransmitters can be altered; their transmission can be disrupted; their binding to receptors can go awry; and their degradation can be inhibited.[776]

What follows is a brief discussion of some of the most harmful metals.

Manganese

Manganese is an essential nutrient. A minute amount is needed from the diet for healthy bones, skin, antioxidant production, and blood sugar control. But larger exposures of manganese are dangerous—another example of a Janus-like substance. Too much manganese triggers a significant drop of protective glutathione in the brain.[777] Manganese mimics calcium and can therefore interfere with normal cell signals.[778]

Manganese poisoning, which usually occurs in welders[779] and miners, results in a Parkinson's-like disorder. But even chronic, low-level exposure of this metal may contribute to PD. In Brescia, northern Italy, the air is polluted from local metal-processing plants. The soot that collects on people's windowsills has been tested; it shows high levels of manganese. Brescia has one of the world's highest rates of PD.[780]

Manganese is also found in pesticides that are linked to PD (such as Maneb). It has been suggested that manganese particles found in vehicle exhaust fumes increase the risk of PD.[781] Manganese is one factor that is believed to contribute to the occurrence of PD in urban areas in America.[782]

Low levels of manganese in air and water are associated with cognitive deficits in children.[783]

Each year, hundreds of tons of manganese are released into the atmosphere in the United States alone.[784]

Lead

Lead disrupts the function of dopamine and also increases the levels of free radicals in the brain. Cumulative lead exposure is associated with PD.[785] Lead is commonly found in paint chips from old homes. But old homes present another danger: the lead solder in plumbing systems may leach into the drinking water. Other sources of lead may include:[786]

➢   polluted air and soil;

➢   cigarettes;

➢   imported pottery;

➢   inexpensive jewelry;

➢   cosmetics (more than 75% of lipsticks contain metals,[787] including lead[788]);

➢   imported canned food;

➢   children's toys.

Mercury

Mercury levels in the body are associated with an increased risk of PD,[789] Alzheimer's Disease,[790] autoimmune diseases, [791] and cardiovascular disease. [792]   Mercury is taken up by the locus coeruleus[793] and is toxic to the BBB.[794] It is believed to trigger excessive levels of glutamate, a neurotransmitter which becomes toxic at high levels.[795] People with certain genetic vulnerabilities are at greater risk for mercury toxicity, resulting in motor and non-motor problems.[796] People with greater than 12 dental amalgams have high levels of mercury in their brains.[797] Mercury can stay in the brain for decades.[798] Besides dental amalgams, sources of mercury include:

➤ fish consumption;

➤ batteries;

➤ light bulbs;

➤ computer parts;

➤ chemical test kits.

Aluminum

Aluminum is the common metal in the environment. It is difficult to avoid it, as it is in the air, soil, and water. But aluminum exposure promotes

PD;[799] high levels of the metal are found in the brains of people with PD.[800] There are several pathways by which aluminum can be disruptive to normal brain functioning: by interfering with iron metabolism; by damaging the BBB; by upsetting normal energy production; and by triggering obesity.[801] Aluminum reduces the number of new nerve cells. This effect is worsened when combined with a high-fat diet.[802]

Aluminum is found in the following products:

➤ Most antacids;

➤ Antiperspirants, lip balms, toothpastes, and cosmetics;

➤ Cheeses, refined table salt, baking powder, and cake mixes (aluminum is added to prevent clumping);

➤ Aluminum wrappers, foil, cookware, and soda cans.

SOLVENTS

Trichloroethylene (TCE) is a great chemical for removing grease. It is found in paint removers, dry-cleaning preparations, and many common household cleaning products. Similar chemicals are perchloroethylene (PERC), carbon tetrachloride (CCl4), toluene, xylene, and n-hexane.

But solvents have a disastrous effect on the human body. TCE significantly reduces the activity of mitochondria, the "powerhouses" of our cells. The effect is especially pronounced in the dopamine producing cells of the substantia nigra.

Can solvents cause PD? In a factory in Kentucky, workers removed grease from machine parts by cleaning them in large vats of TCE. The workers were up to their elbows in the chemical. Not only did the solvent soak through their gloves, but they also breathed in the powerful fumes.

It was discovered that many of the retirees from this company developed PD. An international team of medical investigators did their best to track down former employees; they were eventually able to check the health status of 65 former workers. Each of the former workers had been exposed to TCE for at least 8 years. Some worked at the factory for more than 25 years. Of the 65 factory retirees, 30 had PD.[803]

In another fascinating research project, 99 pairs of twins were studied; one of the twins had developed PD. After detailed questioning about their exposures to chemicals, it was found that the twin who had developed PD generally had a higher exposure to a solvent. For example, exposure to TCE increased the risk of PD by six times. But if there was high exposure to both TCE and PERC, the risk of PD increased *nine times*. [804]

Millions of tons of TCE and related chemicals are released into the environment each year, contaminating the soil, the air, and water supplies, eventually finding their way into our food.[805]

PCBS (POLYCHLORINATED BIPHENYLS)

PCBs are man-made chemicals used as flame-retardants, coolants and insulators in a wide range of industries. PCBs disrupt the BBB;[806] the effect is worse when someone is exposed to PCBs and food toxins.[807] PCBs are banned, but they have a long half-life, which means their effects linger in the environment. There is an association between PCBs and PD, especially in females.[808]

Unfortunately, a chemical used instead of PCBs (called PBDEs, or polybrominated diphenyl ethers) is also damaging to dopamine-producing cells.[809]

PERSISTENT ORGANIC POLLUTANTS

Unfortunately, many pesticides, solvents, and other toxins have polluted the food chain. Moreover, they do not degrade. What this means in that once they get into our bodies, they stay there. Many of these "Persistent Organic Pollutants" (POPs) become stored within our body fat. POPs disrupt our hormonal balances, leading to obesity and a multitude of diseases, including PD.[810] It is believed that the mechanism by which POPs lead to PD is via damage to neuro-transmitter vesicles.[811]

SMOKING

Interestingly, smoking lowers the risk of developing PD.[812] This may be due to the beneficial effects of nicotine. In addition to raising levels of detoxifying enzymes in the brain,[813] nicotine also protects dopamine producing cells,[814] and prevents the misfolding of alpha-synuclein.[815]

However, smoking is linked to the onset of numerous conditions—ranging from cancer to hypertension to other neurodegenerative diseases. This is probably due to the toxins within tobacco.[816] For example, tobacco plants absorb lead, cadmium,[817] and radiation[818] from the soil. Smoking raises blood levels of advanced glycation end-products (AGEs), harman, and norharman[819] (as we discussed in the Diet chapter, these molecules are found in highly processed foods). Smokeless tobacco is also dangerous to the brain.[820]

Overall, the health risks associated with smoking outweigh the anti-PD benefits. The safest way to raise one's levels of nicotine is by eating nicotine-rich foods (see Diet chapter).

DRUG USE

There is an increased risk of PD among drug users.[821] Methamphetamine is a known trigger of the misfolding of alpha-synuclein,[822] as is cocaine.[823] Methamphetamine also damages dopamine vesicles.[824] Men who use methamphetamine raise their risk of PD by three times; women who use it raise their risk of PD by five times.[825]

Marijuana reduces the release of dopamine.[826] Drug abuse alters other shields, such as levels of neurotrophic factors[827] and the release of neurotransmitters.[828] Reminiscent of Dr. Langston's early work with the "frozen addicts," a new generation of drug users exchange "recipes" (on the Internet) for drug formulas. These new illegal drug cocktails also cause PD-like conditions.[829]

RADIATION

There are two types of radiation that we encounter, classified as "ionizing" radiation, and "non-ionizing" radiation. Each of them has the potential to be toxic to the brain.

Ionizing radiation refers to the type of energy that is emitted from X-rays, mammograms, fluoroscopy, CAT scans, and nuclear imaging. Tanning beds also expose people to ionizing radiation.

CAT scans deliver hundreds of times the radiation of a simple dental X-ray. It has been estimated that approximately one-third of CAT scans performed in the United

States each year are unnecessary.[830] It is well known that there are risks of developing cancer due to ionizing radiation exposure (especially in children).[831] It has been hypothesized that it can contribute to the onset of PD and other brain diseases.[832] Virtually every one of our multiple shields can be damaged by radiation toxicity, ranging from the BBB to mitochondria to antioxidant defense mechanisms.[833]

Radon is another source of ionizing radiation. This odorless, colorless gas comes from the natural breakdown of uranium and thorium—two naturally radioactive substances in the soil. Radon can accumulate in homes through cracks in the foundation. In addition to being linked to lung cancer, radon may be considered another "hit" that can result in neurodegeneration. Radon accumulates tenfold in the brain.[834] The Environmental Protection Agency recommends that all homes be tested for radon.

Non-ionizing radiation refers to the exposure from power lines, microwaves, and cell phones. Even though we have come to rely upon our cell phones, there are dangers with its usage. In terms of PD, there are numerous risks with cell phones:

➢ cell phone radiation has the potential to trigger the misfolding of proteins;[835]

➢ it can cause the accumulation of manganese in the brain;[836]

➢ it may stimulate autoimmune diseases;[837]

➢ it lowers levels of melatonin[838] and other antioxidants;[839]

➢ it upsets circadian rhythms, especially when the exposure is at night;[840]

Additional studies on laboratory animals also point to the dangers of cell phone radiation. Rats that had a single 2 hour cell phone exposure had weakening of their Blood-Brain Barriers that lasted for two weeks.[841] Guinea pigs that received twelve hours a day of cell phone exposure had decreased levels of glutathione, a potent brain antioxidant.[842] Rats exposed to cell phone radiation had significantly lower levels of the neurotransmitters dopamine, norepinephrine, and serotonin.[843]

In order to minimize health risks linked to cell phone usage, there are several recommendations:[844]

1. Buy a cell phone with a low Specific Absorption Rate (SAR): the amount of energy absorbed by the body;

2. Whenever possible, send text messages instead of speaking on a cell phone;

3. If you must speak on a cell phone, put it on speakerphone, and make the conversations as brief as possible (long conversations should be made on landlines);

YOUR ACTION PLAN

☞   It is easy to say "avoid exposures to toxins and pollutants" but it is not always easy to implement—we live in a polluted world. Unfortunately, reducing levels of toxins is low on the agenda of politicians, worldwide.[845]

☞   Don't smoke. Don't do drugs.

☞   An important step that you can take is to become more aware of your day-to-day exposures from your environment. Here are some informative websites that can help you to learn more about your environmental exposures:

☞   Air Now, for checking air quality:

http://airnow.gov/

☞   Environmental Health Trust:

http://ehtrust.org/

☞   Toxicology Data Network:

toxnet.nlm.nih.gov

☞   Environmental Working Group:

http://www.ewg.org/

☞   Well-water testing and treatment:

http://www.cdc.gov/healthywater/drinking/private/wells/treatment.html

☞   Choosing a water filter:

http://www.ewg.org/report/ewgs-water-filter-buying-guide

☞ Pesticides-induced Disease Database: http://www.beyondpesticides.org/health/

☞ If you must use pesticides, wear protective clothing. Protective gloves lower the PD risk for most (but not all) pesticides.[846] The proper use of protective clothing while applying pesticides and other chemicals:

http://www.ppp.purdue.edu/Pubs/ppp-38.pdf

☞ Organic gardening:

http://www.organicgardening.com

☞ Understanding the chemical contents of household products:

www.ewg.org/skindeep

☞ Quitting smoking:

http://smokefree.gov/

☞   Resources for drug-addiction treatment:

http://www.drugabuse.gov/publications/princi-ples-drug-addiction-treatment-research-based-guide-third-edition/resources

☞   Recommendations from Dr. Brenner and Dr. Eric Hall, experts in how to minimize exposure to ion-izing radiation: If your doctor orders a CAT scan for you, express your concerns about radiation. Ask if an alternative (such as an MRI or an ultra-sound) is appropriate. Of course, the need for a proper diagnosis may require the use of a CAT scan; in that case, ask the CAT scan technician to use the lowest dose, if possible.

☞   Choose a cell phone with a low Specific Absorp-tion Rate (SAR):

http://sarvalues.com

☞   The Environmental Protection Agency's guide to radon:

http://www.epa.gov/radon

☞   Remember the importance of the other shields: diet, sleep, and exercise. For example, in terms of protecting against radiation, many vegetables have been found to be "radioprotective," especially broccoli, cabbage, and cauliflower.[847] Sleep, with normal levels of melatonin, protects cells against radiation-induced damage.[848]

9

Management of Medical Problems

There are numerous health issues that have the potential of worsening PD. Some of these problems can be prevented through a healthy lifestyle. Regular medical checkups and following medical advice is recommended to lower disease risk.

METABOLIC SYNDROME: THE INFLAMMATORY MIX OF OBESITY, DIABETES, HYPERTENSION, AND MORE

Approximately 70% of adult Americans are either overweight or obese, according to the Centers for Disease Control and Prevention.[849] The numbers are similar in Europe, according to the World Health Organization.[850]

"Metabolic syndrome" is the combination of obesity, insulin resistance, high blood pressure, high triglycerides, and low HDL (high-density lipoproteins). It is also characterized by high levels of inflammation in the body. Metabolic syndrome is a risk factor for developing diabetes (which worsens PD), cardiovascular, and neurodegenerative diseases. It is hypothesized that metabolic syndrome worsens PD in a variety of ways—including mitochondrial abnormalities, increased neuroinflammation, an imbalance of antioxidants, damage to blood vessels, decreased functioning of the vagus nerve,[851] and other mechanisms that throw off our multiple shields.[852]

Fat cells secrete inflammatory chemicals that are extremely harmful. One of them is *Tumor Necrosis Factor alpha*.[853] Let's abbreviate it as TNF. Elevated levels of TNF can be due to obesity, or in response to injuries and diseases. In a deadly cascade of events, high levels of TNF have been shown to trigger neuroinflammation and brain diseases. It is theorized that as neuroinflammation worsens and neurons die, immune cells react in response. When the immune cells die, they release iron; iron promotes the production of free radicals, further damaging neurons, and the cycle feeds on itself.[854] TNF also disrupts normal levels of neurotransmitters, thus setting the stage for PD.[855] In a laboratory experiment, mice exposed to chronically high levels of TNF lost more than 60% of their dopamine-producing cells *within 3 weeks.*[856]

There are many other reasons why metabolic syndrome is dangerous for the brain, including:

➢ Alterations in overall body metabolism: these changes are due not only to fat, but also to the toxins that are stored in the fat cells.[857] Some toxins actually trigger weight gain;[858]

➢ Obesity is linked to altered levels of dopamine release in the brain;[859]

➢ Obesity and high blood pressure cause abnormalities in vital parts of the Blood-Brain Barrier;[860]

➢ Obesity causes dangerous alterations in the hypothalamus, a key component of the Autonomic Nervous System;[861]

➢ It is not uncommon for people with metabolic syndrome to develop sleep apnea.[862] If left untreated, it can cause decreased oxygen to the brain and thereby worsen PD;[863]

➢ With an increase in obesity, brain size decreases.[864]

In summary, avoiding or minimizing metabolic syndrome is an important feature of the anti-PD lifestyle.

AUTOIMMUNE DISEASES

Autoimmune diseases occur when the immune system fails to recognize that the "foreign invader" is not a virus or bacteria; rather, it is the body's own tissue. It has been theorized for many years that PD may be an autoimmune disease, or at least that there is an autoimmune aspect to the disease process.[865] Dr. David Sulzer and his team at Columbia University found that molecules on the surfaces of dopamine neurons can provoke an immune response.[866] This supports the notion that PD is at least partially explained as an autoimmune process. The worsening of an autoimmune disease may worsen PD.

INFECTIONS

For many years, it has been proposed that PD may be due to common infections.[867] Autopsies of some people who died from PD have yielded a fascinating result: a strain of the influenza virus ("the flu") has been found in cells that produce dopamine.[868] In animals, another strain of the flu has been shown to reduce the number of dopamine-producing cells by 17%.[869] Theoretically, this could explain why some people with PD get worse after a bout with the flu.

Some types of influenza can enter the brain through the nasal cavity, disrupt the Autonomic Nervous System, and cause PD or PD-like conditions. Moreover, infections can sensitize the nervous system, making the effects of the pesticide paraquat even more toxic[870]—an example of how the combination of hits lowers the threshold the worsening of PD.

This book is being written during the time of the coronavirus outbreak. Preliminary reports indicate that in addition to affecting the lungs and hearts of those stricken during the pandemic, the nervous system may also be involved. Many of the early symptoms are non-specific, but apparently the central nervous symptom is under significant stress.[871] Time will tell if survivors of the coronavirus develop PD or PD-like conditions.

CHRONIC PAIN

It has been known that people who suffer from chronic pain have neurodegenerative changes (as demonstrated by brain imaging). Chronic pain can also be a pre-clinical problem of PD.[872] But the relationship between pain and brain degeneration is not always clear.

Researchers studied people who suffered from severe hip arthritis. They were scheduled for total hip replacements. All of the patients had chronic, high levels of pain. MRIs of the brain were done prior to their surgeries and six months afterwards. Fortunately, the surgeries essentially eliminated their pain. The follow-up MRIs showed that regions of brain degeneration were substantially reversed after the procedures. The researchers hypothesized that chronic pain messages cause shrinkage of brain regions.[873] Regions of brain degeneration may differ between various painful conditions.[874]

The "pain-brain" connection has additional complexities:

> Inflammation (such as which occurs with arthritis) disrupts the Blood-Brain Barrier;[875]

➤ People in pain tend to become sedentary, which is bad for the brain;

➤ Pain in PD can be "central" (coming from the brain and spinal cord) or peripheral (such as from an arthritic joint), or both. These distinctions are not always addressed by the healthcare team. It is important to discusses this with your providers. There is no need to suffer;

➤ Chronic pain interferes with sleep, and poor sleep adds to pain[876] and poor health. Moreover, some pain medications have an unfortunate side-effect: sleep disturbance;[877]

➤ Vitamin D deficiencies, common in PD, are also linked to both central and peripheral pain conditions.[878]

DENTAL HEALTH

People with PD tend to have unhealthy teeth and gums; it is usually blamed on the movement problems of the disease which limit normal dental care. However, poor oral hygiene may precede the onset of PD.[879]

It is important to brush and floss your teeth regularly, as good dental care lowers the buildup of bacteria called *Streptococcus mutans*.[880] Not only does it cause cavities, but it is also associated with obesity[881] and heart disease.[882] In addition to daily oral hygiene, tea consumption lowers levels of *Streptococcus mutans*.[883]

THE DANGERS OF POLYPHARMACY

"Polypharmacy" refers to taking more than four prescription medications per day. Although some people need multiple medications, the risk of drug interactions rises with more drugs. This is important to our anti-PD lifestyle, as a common mimic of PD is drug-induced Parkinsonism (DIP). Estimates vary as to how often people initially diagnosed with PD are later found to have DIP: somewhere between 7%[884] and as high as 34%.[885] Patients with DIP do not have true PD, but often display many of the typical motor problems of PD. A wide range of medications can cause DIP. The most common are psychiatric medications and antidepressants.[886]

Moreover, for people with PD, some PD medications can cause a heart problem (detected on an electrocardiogram) called long QT syndrome.[887] Dozens of drugs (including some over-the counter medications) can interfere with your PD medications. Long QT syndrome can cause abnormalities of the heart's electrical activity. This can not only lead to feeling unwell; it can also lead to sudden death.

Before taking any new medication or supplement (pre-scribed or over-the counter), discuss it first with your doctor.

YOUR ACTION PLAN

☞   If you have any elements of the metabolic syn-drome, follow the advice of your healthcare team (internist, endocrinologist, dietician, physical therapist, etc.) for proper medical management.

☞   If you have an autoimmune disease, closely follow the advice of your rheumatologist to avoid wors-ening of your disease.

☞   Get a yearly flu shot. In addition, The Centers for Disease Control and Prevention has the following recommendations for preventing the flu: http://www.cdc.gov/flu/about/qa/preventing.htm

☞   If you have chronic pain (such as from severe arthritis), consult with an orthopedist, pain specialist, or neurologist. You may be referred for
physical therapy or acupuncture. There is no need
to suffer if help is available. "Biting the bullet" and
enduring the pain is bad for the brain, and your
emotions.

☞   Take care of your teeth and gums. See your dentist
regularly.

☞   Recommendations to decrease the risks of polypharmacy:[888]

    o   Keep an up-to-date list of all medications,
dosages, frequencies, and reasons why you
are taking them. This includes prescription
medications, over the counter drugs, and
supplements.

    o   Be aware of possible side-effects of your
medications.

    o   If you use multiple physicians, make sure
they are all aware of your medication list,
and of any newly prescribed medications.

Try to use one pharmacy: the pharmacist may be able to spot any "red flags" in terms of high-risk drug interactions.

☞ Remember the positive, synergistic effects of the multiple shields: good nutrition/a healthy gut; stress reduction; good sleep; and non-exhaustive exercise. These factors are anti-inflammatory and can help to fight the effects of the metabolic syndrome and autoimmune diseases. Exercise also strengthens the immune system and provides protection against infections.[889]

10

Preventing Head Injuries

Any type of trauma to the head is dangerous. The injury could be due to physical contact, such as what occurs with a fall or with a blow to the head. It could also occur when the brain moves rapidly within the skull (which can occur with a motor vehicle accident/whiplash injury). More than 1.7 million people suffer head trauma each year in America.[890] For a person with PD, a head injury can be a major setback and significantly worsen their quality of life.

 A head injury, also called a traumatic brain injury (TBI), disrupts the normal functioning of the brain and results in the loss of brain cells. It is well known that a mild TBI (such as a concussion) can result in balance problems, difficulty concentrating, and altered sleep patterns.[891] But even lower impact blows to the head can take their toll.

Within 100 milliseconds of a traumatic brain injury, the following pathological processes may occur:[892]

> Damage to the Blood-Brain Barrier (BBB).[893] Moreover, the BBB becomes inflamed, which results in additional physical pressure and biochemical insult to the BBB and neurons ("secondary brain damage");[894]

> From the initial event, destruction of neurons; this also triggers secondary brain damage;

> Significant, sometimes life-threatening, alterations in blood flow to the brain;[895]

> Neurotransmitter loss. In experimental models with rats, serious head trauma resulted in a 15% loss of dopamine-producing cells shortly after the injury. But the damage did not stop there. Norepinephrine levels dropped for a week.[896] Dopamine-producing cells continued to be lost for 6 months after the trauma, resulting in a final 30% loss of dopamine-producing cells. Moreover, dopamine-producing cells became more vulnerable to toxins for months after the occurrence of the trauma.[897] Based on these losses of dopamine-

producing cells, we can understand why a person with PD (who already has low levels of dopamine) who suffers a head injury would not fare well.

➤ Disruption of levels of potassium, calcium, and glucose metabolism in the brain;[898]

➤ Massive increases in free-radical production. In certain animal models, it has been demonstrated that free-radicals can increase by as much as 250% after head trauma;[899]

➤ In an animal model of a TBI, alpha-synuclein was detected in dopamine-producing cells 60 days after the injury;[900]

➤ Because of the communication between the brain and other organs (via the vagus nerve and the Autonomic Nervous System), brain damage caused by a TBI can also result in cardiac and gastrointestinal problems.[901] Increased intestinal permeability—a "leaky gut"— can begin within hours of a TBI.[902] The normal functioning of the vagus nerve is diminished after a TBI.[903]

THE MAJOR CAUSES OF TRAUMATIC BRAIN INJURIES

Among civilians (in other words, non-military), falls represent the number one cause of TBIs.[904] More than 60% of TBIs over the age of 65 are due to falls.

Falling is a major problem in PD. On average, 60% of PD patients have reported falling once, and 39% report falling more than once. The average of repeated falls per year is reported to be more than 20 times.[905] Of course, not every fall injures the head, but the potential is there.

Other causes of TBIs:

➤ Motor vehicle accidents and traffic related events (more than 17% of TBIs);

➤ Assaults account for roughly 10% of TBIs.

YOUR ACTION PLAN

A TBI can occur in a split second. But there are things that can be done to decrease your risk:[906]

☞   Reducing the risk of TBIs due to falls in older adults:

    o   If you are taking any medications that cause dizziness, discuss it with your doctor. There may be a different medication, dosage, or timing to decrease your dizziness;

    o   If your vision is a problem, see your eye-care professional;

    o   If you have weakness and/or balance problems, see a physical therapist. Corrective exercises can be beneficial;

    o   Have a home safety evaluation, performed by a physical therapist, occupational therapist, or registered nurse. A home safety evaluation can spot places where a fall may occur. The healthcare professional can make recommendations to rectify the situation. Simple steps, such as removing clutter, using a nightlight, or installing grab bars in the bathroom can prevent a fall.

☞ Reducing the risk of TBIs due to motor vehicle accidents:

  ○   wear your seat belt;

  ○   do not drive while impaired;

  ○   do not text and drive, and drive defensively;

  ○   pedestrians need to be vigilant when crossing the street.

☞ Reducing the risk of TBIs due to assaults: A person may be assaulted during a crime, such as during a robbery. But many cases of assault are perpetrated by abusive family members. The CDC has extensive resources for dealing with the subject of violence prevention:
http://www.cdc.gov/violenceprevention/

11

Quality of Life with PD

Dealing with PD can be a daunting task. How can one still live "a good life" with PD? "Quality of Life" (QoL) has been studied in PD patients worldwide, and certain conclusions can be drawn.

Although worsening of any PD-related issue can cause distress and potentially worsen one's QoL, there are some points that appear to be similar in people with PD regardless of their age, male or female, or where they live.

The factors that improve QoL include all of the topics contained within this book, such as nutrition, mobility, and management of non-motor issues. A good healthcare team can help you to deal with any new problems that may arise.

The most-reported movement factors that impair QoL include:

➢   dyskinesias (usually related to medication levels);[907]

➢   motor fluctuations (on-off);[908]

➢   muscle rigidity (especially in the trunk).[909]

The non-motor factors that impair QoL include:

➢   worsening of sleep;[910]

➢   cognitive loss;

➢   anxiety;

➢   depression;[911]

➢   hallucinations;

➢   constipation/gastrointestinal symptoms;

➢   urinary problems;

➢   fatigue;

➢   drops in blood pressure;

> ➢   excessive perspiration.912

It is recommended that you pay special attention to these areas of your life, and do not hesitate to discuss them with your doctor if you feel that your QoL is suffering.

Interestingly, a recent study found that a decreased QoL due to many of these issues can at least be partially reversed with an improvement in nutritional status, with regular monitoring by caregivers and members of the healthcare team.[913]

It is always important to keep in mind that your care needs to be centered around you, and not just based on decisions made predominantly by your doctor. Your care needs to be a partnership between the doctor and the patient/caregiver. Ideally, all directions of your care need to be based on shared decision making.[914]

Before going to the doctor (or having a telehealth session), you and your caregiver should have any questions or concerns written out. It is acceptable to bring pages printed out from "Dr. Google" or from other patient education materials. Enhancing your own health literacy is not only important for you to advance your knowledge of PD, but also to show your medical team that you are taking an active role in your care. Health literacy—

defined as the ability to obtain, understand, and communicate basic health information—is a skill held by
only 12% of the population.[915]

Another strategy, when discussing problems with your
doctor (or with other members of the healthcare team),
is to ask the question, "I know this can be blamed on my
PD, but could it be something else?" It is always possible
that your problem could be due to a non-PD condition
which is potentially treatable. Case in point: one of my
patients repeatedly complained to his doctor of low back
pain and difficulty urinating. His doctor consistently re-
plied," Remember, you have Parkinson's. These com-
plaints are because of your condition. You just have to
accept it." The real picture emerged when the patient began urinating blood and was rushed to the emergency
room. A simple X-ray revealed that the patient had a kidney tumor, completely unrelated to his PD. Removal of
the tumor eliminated both his urinary problem and his
back pain.

Being an active patient—someone who is actively participating in one's care, with the assistance of a caregiver—
is vital for personalizing your Parkinson's Disease care.

Please feel free to e-mail me with comments and questions:

<Benweinstock@gmail.com>

Index

Endnotes

[1] Titova N, Chaudhuri KR. Personalzied Medicine in Parkinson's Disease: Time to Be Precise. Movement Disorders, Vol. 32, No. 8, 2017, p. 1147-1154.

[2] "Statistics on Parkinson's." http://www.pdf.org/en/parkinson_statistics Accessed October 3, 2014.

[3] Tanner CM, Marder K. "Movement Disorders," in Neuroepidemiology: From Principles to Practice, Oxford, 2004, p. 133.

[4] "Statistics on Parkinson's." http://www.pdf.org/en/parkinson_statistics Accessed October 3, 2014.

[5] Marras C, Lang A. Parkinson's disease subtypes: lost in translation? J Neurol Neurosurg Psychiatry, 2013; 84; p. 409–415.

[6] https://www.ajmc.com/focus-of-the-week/poll-finds-1-in-4-people-with-parkinson-disease-misdiagnosed . Accessed January 12, 2020.

[7] Adler CH, et al. Low clinical diagnostic accuracy of early vs advanced Parkinson disease. Neurology, 2014, 83:406–412.

[8] https://parkinsonsnewstoday.com/parkinsons-disease-tests-diagnosis/datscan/. Accessed January 12, 2020.

[9] https://www.mayoclinic.org/medical-professionals/neurology-neurosurgery/news/tissue-biopsy-for-identifying-early-parkinsons/mac-20431299. Accessed January 12, 2020.

[10] http://www.pdf.org/en/parkinson_statistics . Accessed July 16, 2013.

[11] Dorsey ER, et al, Projected number of people with Parkinson disease in the most populous nations, 2005 through 2030. Neurology, 2007; 68(5); p. 384-386.

[12] Tanner CM, What Causes Parkinson's Disease? An Epidemiologists Perspective, 2013 Symposium Videos, 7th Annual Parkinson's Disease Symposium. http://www.youtube.com/watch?v=txzXaeAghOA Accessed April 17, 2014.

[13] Collier TJ, Kanaan NM, Kordower JH. Ageing as a primary risk factor for Parkinson's disease: evidence from studies of non-human primates. Nat Rev Neurosci. 2011; 12(6): p. 359–366.

[14] Klepac N, et al. An update on the management of young-onset Parkinson's disease. Degenerative Neurological and Neuromuscular Disease 2013;3; p. 53–62.

[15] Van Den Eeden SK, et al. Incidence of Parkinson's Disease: Variation by Age, Gender, and Race/Ethnicity. Am. J. Epidemiol. 2003;157 (11); p. 1015-1022.

[16] De Rijk MC, et al. Neurologic Diseases in the Elderly Research Group Prevalence of Parkinson's disease in Europe: A collaborative study of population-based cohorts. Neurology. 2000;54(11 Suppl 5); p.S21–S23.

[17] Schultz W. Reward Signaling by Dopamine Neurons. Neuroscientist, 2001; 7; p. 293-302.

[18] Peters R. Ageing and the brain. Postgrad Med J 2006;82; p. 84–88.

[19] Buchman AS, et al. Locus Coeruleus Neuron Density and Parkinsonism in Older Adults without Parkinson's Disease. Mov Disorders, 2012; 27(13); p.1625–1631.

[20] Carvey PM, Punati A, Newman MB. Progressive dopamine neuron loss in Parkinson's disease: the multiple hit hypothesis. Cell Transplant. 2006;15(3); p.239-250.

[21] Nelson LM. Military Service and Parkinson's Disease. 2013. Prepared for: U.S. Army Medical Research and Materiel Command, Fort Detrick, Maryland 21702-5012.

[22] Gibbered FB, Simmonds JP. Neurological disease in ex-Far-East prisoners of war. The Lancet, 1980; Volume 316, Issue 8186; p. 135–137.

[23] Robson D, Welch E, Beeching NJ, Gill GV. Consequences of captivity: health effects of far East imprisonment in World War II. Q J Med, 2009; 102; p. 87–96.

[24] Tanner CM, Goldman SM, Ross GW, Grate SJ. The disease intersection of susceptibility and exposure: chemical exposures and neurodegenerative disease risk. Alzheimers Dement. 2014;10(3 Suppl); p.S213-25.

[25] Husain AM, Miller PP, Carwile ST. Rem sleep behavior disorder: potential relationship to post-traumatic stress disorder. J Clin Neurophysiol. 2001;18(2); p.148-157.

[26] Swinkels CM, et al. The Association of Sleep Duration, Mental Health, and Health Risk Behaviors among U.S. Afghanistan/Iraq Era Veterans. SLEEP, 2013; Vol. 36, No. 7; p.1019-1025.

[27] Marques O, Outeiro TF. Alpha-synuclein: from secretion to dysfunction and death. Cell Death and Disease, 2012; 3; e350; doi: 10.1.1038/cddis.2012.94

[28] Pifl C, et al. Is Parkinson's disease a vesicular dopamine storage disorder? Evidence from a study in isolated synaptic vesicles of human and nonhuman primate striatum. J Neurosci. 2014 Jun 11;34(24):8210-8. doi: 10.1523/JNEUROSCI.5456-13.2014.

[29] Pacheco C, Aguayo LG, Opazo C. An extracellular mechanism that can explain the neurotoxic effects of alpha-synuclein aggregates in the brain. Frontiers in Physiology, 2012; Volume 3, Article 297; 10 pages.

[30] Stefanoni G, et al. Alpha-Synuclein, Oxidative Stress and Autophagy Failure: Dangerous Liaisons in Dopaminergic Neurodegeneration. In: Etiology and Pathophysiology of Parkinson's Disease, edited by Abdul Qayyum Rana, ISBN 978-953-307-462-7, Published: October 12, 2011 under CC BY 3.0 license.

[31] Bousset L, et al. Structural and functional characterization of two alpha-synuclein strains. Nature Communications, 2013; 4, Article number: 2575; doi:10.1038/ncomms3575

[32] Tonges L, et al. Alpha-synuclein mutations impair axonal regeneration in models of Parkinson's disease. Front. Aging Neurosci., 2014; doi: 10.3389/fnagi.2014.00239

[33] Prabhakaran K, Chapman GD, Gunasekar PG. α-Synuclein overexpression enhances manganese-induced neurotoxicity through the NF-κB-mediated pathway. Toxicol Mech Methods. 2011;21(6); p.435-443.

[34] Braak H, et al. Staging of brain pathology related to sporadic Parkinson's disease. Neurobiol Aging, 2003;24(2); p.197-211.

[35] Visanji NP, Brooks PL, Hazrati LN, Lang AE. The prion hypothesis in Parkinson's disease: Braak to the future. Acta Neuropathologica Communications, 2013; 1:2; 12 pages.

[36] Olanow WC, Brundin P. Parkinson's Disease and Alpha Synuclein: Is Parkinson's Disease a Prion-Like Disorder? Movement Disorders Special Issue: The Vatican Conference on Neuroprotection in Parkinson's Disease, 2013; Volume 28, Issue 1; p. 31–40.

[37] Kalaitzakis ME, et al. The dorsal motor nucleus of the vagus is not an obligatory trigger site of Parkinson's disease: a critical analysis of alpha-synuclein staging. Neuropathol Appl Neurobiol 2008;34; p. 284-295.

[38] Weiner WJ. There Is No Parkinson Disease. Archives of Neurology, 2008; Vol. 65, No. 6; p. 706-708.

[39] Monteiro A, Massano J. Parkinson's disease cluster: the wind of change. International Journal of Clinical Neurosciences and Mental Health, 2014; 1;7.

[40] Kordower JH, et al. Disease duration and the integrity of the nigrostriatal system in Parkinson's disease. Brain 2013; 136; p. 2419–2431.

[41] Savica R, Rocca WA, Ahlskog JE. When Does Parkinson Disease Start? Archives of Neurology, 2010;67(7); p. 798-801.

[42] Albin RL, Dauer T. Magic shotgun for Parkinson's disease? Brain, 2014; 137 (5); p. 1274-1275.

[43] Garelick MG, Kennedy BK. TOR on the Brain. Exp Gerontol., 2011; 46(2-3); p. 155–163.

[44] Levy OA, Malagelada C, Greene LA. Cell death pathways in Parkinson's disease: proximal triggers, distal effectors, and final steps. Apoptosis, 2009;14(4); p.478-500.

[45] Adamczyk A, Strosznajder JB. Alpha-synuclein potentiates Ca2+ influx through voltage-dependent Ca2+ channels. Molecular Neuroscience, 2006; Volume 17, Issue 18; p. 1883-1886.

[46] Predinger RDS, et al. Intranasal Administration of Neurotoxicants in Animals: Support for the Olfactory Vector Hypothesis of Parkinson's Disease. Neurotoxicity Research, 2012; Volume 21, Issue 1; p. 90-116.

[47] Ubeda-Banon I, et al. Alpha-Synuclein in the olfactory system in Parkinson's disease: role of neural connections on spreading pathology. Brain Struct Funct. 2013; PMID: 24135772.

[48] Clos AL, Kayed R, Lasagna-Reeves CA. Association of skin with the pathogenesis and treatment of neurodegenerative amyloidosis. Front Neurol. 2012; 3:5. doi: 10.3389/fneur.2012.00005. eCollection 2012.

[49] Kortekaas R, et al. Blood–Brain Barrier Dysfunction in Parkinsonian Midbrain In Vivo. Ann Neurol., 2005; 57; p.176–179.

[50] Zlokovic BV. The Blood-Brain Barrier in Health and Chronic Neurodegenerative Disorders. Neuron, 2008; 57; p. 178-201.

[51] Ibid.

[52] Ibid.

[53] Farkas E, et al. Similar Ultrastructural Breakdown of Cerebrocortical Capillaries in Alzheimer's Disease, Parkinson's Disease, and Experimental Hypertension: What is the Functional Link? Annals of the New York Academy of Sciences, 2000, Volume 903, Vascular Functions in Alzheimer's Disease, p. 72–82.

[54] Maise K, editor. Neurovascular Medicine: Pursuing Cellular Longevity for Healthy Aging. Oxford University Press, 2009, p. 377.

[55] Quaegebeur A , Segura I, Carmeliet P. Pericytes: blood-brain barrier safeguards against neurodegeneration? Neuron. 2010;68(3);p. 321-323.

[56] Sharma HS, Westman J, editors. Blood-Spinal and Brain Barriers in Health and Disease. Elsevier Academic Press, 2004, p. 235.

[57] Oldendorf, WH, Cornford, ME, Brown, WJ. The large apparent work capability of the blood-brain barrier: A study of the mitochondrial content of capillary endothelial cells in brain and other tissues of the rat. Ann Neurol., 1977; 1; p.409–417.

[58] A comparison of the BBB to a medieval castle in terms of immune function is found in: Muldoon LL, et al. Immunologic privilege in the central nervous system and the blood-brain barrier. Journal of Cerebral Blood Flow and Metabolism, 2012, p. 1-9.

[59] Davson H, Oldendorf WH. Transport in the central nervous system. Proceedings of the Royal Society of London, 1967; volume 60, p. 326-329.

[60] Sanchez-Guajardo v, Barnum CJ, Tansey MG, Romero-Ramos M. Neuroimmunological processes in Parkinson's disease and their relation to alpha-synuclein: microglia as the referee between neuronal processes and peripheral immunity. American Society for Neurochemistry, 2013; Volume 5 (2); p. 113-139.

[61] Tang JP, Xu ZQ, Douglas FL, Rakhit A, Melethil S. Increased blood-brain barrier permeability of amino acids in chronic hypertension. Life Sci. 1993;53(25):p. PL417-420.

[62] Yokel RA. Manganese Flux Across the Blood–Brain Barrier. NeuroMolecular Medicine, 2009; Volume 11, Issue 4; p. 297-310.

[63] Zecca L, et al. A proposed dual role of neuromelanin in the pathogenesis of Parkinson's disease. Neurology 2006;67(Suppl 2):S8–S11

[64] Lucchini, R, Zimmerman, N. Lifetime cumulative exposure as a threat for neurodegeneration: Need for prevention strategies on a global scale. Neurotoxicology, 2009; 30; p. 1144-1148.

[65] Kalaria RN, Stockmeier CA, Harik SI. Brain microvessels are innervated by locus ceruleus noradrenergic neurons. Neuroscience Letters, 1989; Volume 97, Issues 1–2; p. 203–208.

[66] Heneka MT, et al. Locus ceruleus controls Alzheimer's disease pathology by modulating microglial functions through norepinephrine. Proc Natl Acad Sci U S A. 2010;107(13); p.6058-6063.

[67] Harik SI, McGunigal T Jr. The protective influence of the locus ceruleus on the blood-brain barrier. Ann Neurol. 1984;15(6); p.568-574.

[68] Kalinin S, et al. Noradrenaline deficiency in brain increases beta-amyloid plaque burden in an animal model of Alzheimer's disease. Neurobiol Aging. 2007; 28(8); p.1206-1214.

[69] Del Tredici K, Braak H. Dysfunction of the locus coeruleus–norepinephrine system and related circuitry in Parkinson's disease-related dementia. J Neurol Neurosurg Psychiatry doi:10.1136/jnnp-2011-301817

[70] Vazey EM, Ashton-Jones G. The emerging role of norepinephrine in cognitive dysfunctions of Parkinson's disease. Front Behav Neurosci. 2012 Jul 25;6:48. doi: 10.3389/fnbeh.2012.00048. eCollection 2012.

[71] LeWitt PA. Norepinephrine: the next therapeutics frontier for Parkinson's disease. Translational Neurodegeneration 2012, 1:4.

[72] Ritz BR, et al. Dopamine transporter genetic variants and pesticides in Parkinson's disease. Environ Health Perspect. 2009;117(6); p.964-969.

[73] Szot P, et al. Sequential Loss of LC Noradrenergic and Dopaminergic Neurons Results in a Correlation of Dopaminergic Neuronal Number to Striatal Dopamine Concentration. Front Pharmacol. 2012; 3:184. doi: 10.3389/fphar.2012.00184. eCollection 2012.

[74] Bennett L, Yang M, Enikolopov G, Iacovitti L. Circumventricular organs: a novel site of neural stem cells in the adult brain. Mol Cell Neurosci., 2009;41(3); p.337-347.

[75] Price MT, Olney JW, Lowry OH, Buchsbaum S. Uptake of exogenous glutamate and aspartate by circumventricular organs but not other regions of brain. J Neurochem., 1981;36(5); p.1774-1780.

[76] Rea WJ, Patel K. Reversibility of Chronic Degenerative Disease and Hypersensitivity: Regulating Mechanisms of Chemical Sensitivity, Volume 1, 2010, CRC Press, page 261.

[77] Ferrari CC, Tarelli R. Parkinson's Disease and Systemic Inflammation. Parkinson's Disease, 2011; Article ID 436813, 9 pages; doi:10.4061/2011/436813

[78] Goldstein DS, Adrenaline and the Inner World. The Johns Hopkins University Press, Baltimore, 2006, p. 8-29. See also: Goldstein DS, Bentho O, Park MY, Sharabi Y. LF power of heart rate variability is not a measure of cardiac sympathetic tone but may be a measure of modulation of cardiac autonomic outflows by baroreflexes. Exp Physiol., 2011; 96(12); p. 1255–1261.

[79] Surmeier DJ, Sulzer D. The pathology roadmap in Parkinson disease. Prion, 2013, 7:1; p. 85–91.

[80] Forsyth CB, et al. Increased Intestinal Permeability Correlates with Sigmoid Mucosa alpha-Synuclein Staining and Endotoxin Exposure Markers in Early Parkinson's Disease. PLoS ONE, 2011; Volume 6, Issue 12; e28032, 10 pages.

[81] Yehuda S, Rabinovitz S, Carasso RL, Mostofsky DI. The role of polyunsaturated fatty acids in restoring the aging neuronal membrane. Neurobiol Aging, 2002;23(5); p.843-853.

[82] McBride HM, Neuspiel M, Wasiak S. Mitochondria: more than just a powerhouse. Curr Biol., 2006;16(14); p.R551-60.

[83] Klecker T, Böckler S, Westermann B. Making connections: interorganelle contacts orchestrate mitochondrial behavior. Trends Cell Biol., 2014;24(9); p.537-545.

[84] Mercado G, Valdés P, Hetz C. An ERcentric view of Parkinson's disease. Trends Mol Med. 2013;19(3); p.165-175.

[85] Aridon P, et al. Protective Role of Heat Shock Proteins in Parkinson's Disease. Neurodegenerative Dis., 2010; DOI: 10.1159/000321548

[86] McNaught KS, Perl DP, Brownell AL, Olanow CW. Systematic exposure to proteasome inhibitors causes a progressive model of Parkinson's disease. Ann. Neurol., 2004; 56 (1); p. 149-162.

[87] Lum MA, et al. Heat shock proteins regulate activation-induced proteasomal degradation of the mature phosphorylated form of protein kinase C. J Biol Chem., 2013;288(38); p.27112-27127.

[88] Yang F, et al. Crosstalk between the proteasome system and autophagy in the clearance of α-synuclein. Acta Pharmacologica Sinica, 2013;34; p. 674–680

[89] Korolchuk VI, Mansilla A, Menzies FM, Rubinsztein DC. Autophagy inhibition compromises degradation of ubiquitin-proteasome pathway substrates. Mol Cell., 2009;33(4); p.517-527.

[90] Pan T, Kondo S, Le W, Jankovic J. The role of autophagy-lysosome pathway in neurodegeneration associated with Parkinson's disease. Brain, 2008;131(Pt 8); p.1969-1978.

[91] Bourdenx M, Bezard E, Dehay B. Lysosomes and α-synuclein form a dangerous duet leading to neuronal cell death. Front Neuroanat., 2014;8:83. doi: 10.3389/fnana.2014.00083. eCollection 2014.

[92] Tatsuta T, Langer T. Quality control of mitochondria: protection against neuro-degeneration and ageing. The EMBO Jornal, 2008; 27; p. 306-314.

[93] Swerdlow RH. Role and Treatment of Mitochondrial DNA-Related Mitochon-drial Dysfunction in Sporadic Neurodegenerative Diseases. Curr Pharm Des., 2011; 17(31); p. 3356–3373.

[94] Bourdenx M, Dehay B, Bezard E. Down-Regulating alpha-Synuclein for Treat-ing Synucleopathies. Movement Disorders, 2014; Vol. 29, No. 12; p. 1463-1465.

[95] Hayashita-Kinoh, et al. Down-regulation of α-synuclein expression can rescue dopaminergic cells from cell death in the substantia nigra of Parkinson's disease rat model. Biochemical and Biophysical Research Communications, 2006; Volume 341, Issue 4; p. 1088–1095.

[96] Andersson U, Tracey KJ. Neural reflexes in inflammation and immunity. J. Exp. Med., 2012; Vol. 209, No. 6; p. 1057-1068.

[97] Andersson U, Tracey KJ. Neural reflexes in inflammation and immunity. J. Exp. Med., 2012; Vol. 209, No. 6; p. 1057-1068.

[98] Ziomber A, et al. Chronic impairment of the vagus nerve function leads to inhi-bition of dopamine but not serotonin neurons in rat brain structures. Pharmacolog-ical Reports, 2012; 64; p. 1359-1367.

[99] Revesz D, et al. Effects of vagus nerve stimulation on rat hippocampal progenitor proliferation. Experimental Neurology, 2008; Volume 214, Issue 2; p. 259-265.

[100] Miwa H, Kubo T, Suzuki A, Kondo T. Intragastric proteasome inhibition in-duces alpha-synuclein-immunopositive aggregations in neurons in the dorsal motor nucleus of the vagus in rats. Neurosci. Lett., 2006, 401 (1-2); p. 146-149.

[101] Braak H, Rüb U, Gai WP, Del Tredici K. Idiopathic Parkinson's disease: possi-ble routes by which vulnerable neuronal types may be subject to neuroinvasion by an unknown pathogen. J Neural Transm., 2003;110(5); p.517-536.

[102] Pavlov VA, Tracey KJ. The vagus nerve and the inflammatory reflex—linking immunity and metabolism. Nat. Rev. Endocrinol., 2012; 8 (12); p. 743-754.

[103] Lotze MT, Tracey KJ. High-mobility group box 1 protein (HMGB1): nuclear weapon in the immune arsenal. Nature Reviews Immunology, 2005; 5; p. 331-342.

[104] Ko EA, Min HJ, Shin JS. Interaction of High Mobility Group Box-1 (HMGB1) with α-synuclein and its aggregation. The Journal of Immunology, 2012; 188; 172.28.

[105] Metz CN, Tracey KJ. It takes nerve to dampen inflammation. Nat Immunol., 2005;6(8); p.756-757.

[106] Payami H, Larsen K, Bernard S, Nutt J. Increased risk of Parkinson's disease in parents and siblings of patients. Annals of Neurology, 36; p. 659–661.

[107] Sveinbjornsdottir S, et al. Familial aggregation of Parkinson's Disease in Iceland. New England Journal of Medicine, 2000; Vol.343, Number 24; p. 1765-1770.

[108] Marder K, et al. Risk of Parkinson's disease among first-degree relatives: A community-based study. Neurology, 1996;47(1); p.155-160.

[109] Nuytemans K, et al. Genetic Etiology of Parkinson Disease Associated with Mutations in the SNCA, PARK2, PINK1, PARK7, and LRRK2 Genes: A Mutation Update. Human Mutation, 2010; Vol. 31, No. 7; p. 763-780.

[110] Burbulla LF, Krüger R. Converging environmental and genetic pathways in the pathogenesis of Parkinson's disease. J Neurol Sci., 2011;306(1-2); p.1-8.

[111] Soreq L, et al. Meta-analysis of genetic and environmental Parkinson's disease models reveals a common role of mitochondrial protection pathways. Neurobiol Dis. 2012;45(3); p. 1018-1030.

[112] Olden K, White SL. Health-related disparities: influence of environmental factors. Med Clin North Am., 2005; 89(4); p. 721-738.

[113] Iraola-Guzmán S, Estivill X, Rabionet R. DNA methylation in neurodegenerative disorders: a missing link between genome and environment? Clinical Genetics, 2011; Volume 80, Issue 1; p. 1–14.

[114] Herbert RM. Everyday Epigenetics: From Molecular Intervention to Public Health and Lifestyle Medicine. North American Journal of Medicine and Science, 2013; Vol. 6, No.3; p. 167-170.

[115] Shawky, RM. Reduced penetrance in human inherited disease. The Egyptian Journal of Medical Human Genetics, 2014; 15; p. 103–111.

[116] Tanner CM, et al. Parkinson Disease in Twins: an etiologic study. JAMA, 1999; Vol. 281, No. 4; p. 341-346.

[117] Goldman S, et al. Solvent Exposures and Parkinson's Disease Risk in Twins. Annals of Neurology, 2012; Volume 71, Issue 6; p. 776–784.

[118] Lim U, Song MA. Dietary and lifestyle factors of DNA methylation. Methods Mol Biol. 2012;863; p.359-376.

[119] Masliah E, Dumaop W, Galasko D, Desplats P. Distinctive patterns of DNA methylation associated with Parkinson disease. Epigenetics, 2013; Volume 8, Issue 10; p. 1030-1038.

[120] Mouradian MM. MicroRNAs in Parkinson's disease. Neurobiol Dis., 2012;46(2); p.279-284.

[121] Tarallo S, et al. MicroRNA expression in relation to different dietary habits: a comparison in stool and plasma samples. Mutagenesis, 2014; 29 (5); p. 385-391.

[122] Nielson S, et al. The miRNA Plasma Signature in Response to Acute Aerobic Exercise and Endurance Training. PLOS ONE, 2014; DOI: 10.1371/journal.pone.0087308.

[123] Davis CJ, Bohnet SG, Meyerson JM, Krueger JM. Sleep loss changes microRNA levels in the brain: a possible mechanism for state-dependent translational regulation. Neurosci Lett.,2007;422(1); p.68-73

[124] Cui Y, et al. Differential expression of miRNA in rat myocardial tissues under psychological and physical stress. Experimental and Therapeutic Medicine, 2014. DOI: 10.3892/etm.2014.1504

[125] LeRoith D. microRNAs: What the Clinician Should Know About This New Frontier. Diabetes Care, 2014;37; p.1176–1177.

[126] Saunders-Pullman R, et al. Progression in the LRRK2-Asssociated Parkinson Disease Population. JAMA Neurol. 2018 Mar 1;75(3):312-319.

[127] Mata IF, et al. LRRK2 in Parkinson's disease: protein domains and functional insights. TRENDS in Neurosciences, 2006; Vol.29, No.5; p. 286-293.

[128] Bailey RM, et al. LRRK2 phosphorylates novel tau epitopes and promotes tauopathy. Acta Neuropathologica, 2013, 126(6); p. 809-827.

[129] Bravo-San Pedro JM, et al. Parkinson's disease: leucine-rich repeat kinase 2 and autophagy, intimate enemies. Parkinsons Dis. 2012; 2012:151039. doi: 10.1155/2012/151039.

[130] Orenstein S, et al. Interplay of LRRK2 with chaperone-mediated autophagy. Nature Neuroscience, 2013; 16; p. 394–406.

[131] Greggio E, Civiero L, Bisaglia M, Bubacco L. Parkinson's disease and immune system: is the culprit LRRKing in the periphery? Journal of Neuroinflammation, 2012; 9:94; p. 1-7.

[132] Goldwurm S, et al. Evaluation of LRRK2 G2019S penetrance: Relevance for genetic counseling in Parkinson disease. Neurology, 2007; vol. 68 no. 14; p. 1141-1143.

[133] Desplats P, et al. Combined exposure to Maneb and Paraquat alters transcriptional regulation of neurogenesis-related genes in mice models of Parkinson's disease. Mol. Neurodegener. 2012; 7: 49. Published online Sep 28, 2012. doi: 10.1186/1750-1326-7-49.

[134] Lashuel HA, Overk CR, Oueslati A, Masliah E. The many faces of α-synuclein: from structure and toxicity to therapeutic target. Nature Reviews Neuroscience, 2013; 14; p. 38-48.

[135] Chung SJ, et al. Alpha-synuclein repeat variants and survival in Parkinson's disease. Movement Disorders, 2014; Volume 29, Issue 8; p. 1053–1057.

[136] Ren H, et al; DJ-1, a cancer and Parkinson's disease associated protein, regulates autophagy through JNK pathway in cancer cells. Cancer Letters, 2010; Volume 297, Issue 1; p. 101–108.

[137] Ariga H, et al. Neuroprotective Function of DJ-1 in Parkinson's Disease. Oxidative Medicine and Cellular Longevity
Volume 2013, Article ID 683920, 9 pages.

[138] Xu X, Martin F, Friedman JS. The familial Parkinson's disease gene DJ-1 (PARK7) is expressed in red cells and plays a role in protection against oxidative damage. Blood Cells Mol Dis., 2010 45(3); p. 227-332.

[139] Bjorkblom B, et al. Parkinson disease protein DJ-1 binds metals and protects against metal-induced cytotoxicity. J Biol Chem. 2013; 288(31); p. 22809-22820.

[140] Amo T, et al. Mitochondrial membrane potential decrease caused by loss of PINK1 is not due to proton leak, but to respiratory chain defects. Neurobiology of Disease 2011; Volume 41, Issue 1; p. 111–118.

[141] Duplan E, et al. ER-stress-associated functional link between Parkin and DJ-1 via a transcriptional cascade involving the tumor suppressor p53 and the spliced X-box binding protein XBP-1. J Cell Sci. 2013; 126(Pt 9); p.2124-2133.

[142] Um, JW, et al. Parkin Directly Modulates 26S Proteasome Activity. The Journal of Neuroscience, 2010; 30(35); p.11805–11814.

[143] Ahmed I, et al. Association between Parkinson's disease and the HLA-DRB1 locus. Mov Disord. 2012; 27(9); p. 1104-1110.

[144] Gerecke KM, Jiao Y, Pagala V, Smeyne RJ. Exercise Does Not Protect against MPTP-Induced Neurotoxicity in BDNF Happloinsufficent Mice. PLOS One, 2012; DOI: 10.1371/journal.pone.0043250

[145] Karamohamed S, et al. BDNF genetic variants are associated with onset age of familial Parkinson disease: GenePD Study. Neurology, 2005;65(11); p:1823-1825.

[146] Elbaz A, et al. Independent and joint effects of the MAPT and SNCA genes in Parkinson's disease. Ann Neurol. 2011; 69(5); p. 778–792.

[147] Gregorio ML, et al. Impact of Genetic Variants of Apolipoprotein E on Lipid Profile in Patients with Parkinson's Disease. BioMed Research International, Volume 2013, Article ID 641515, 7 pages.

[148] Antony PMA, Diedrich NJ, Kruger R, Balling R. The hallmarks of Parkinson's disease. FEBS Journal, 2013; 280(23); p.5981-5993.

[149] Bae EJ, et al. Glucocerebrosidase depletion enhances cell-to-cell transmission of α-synuclein. Nat Commun., 2014;5:4755. doi: 10.1038/ncomms5755.

[150] Bras J, et al. Mutation of the parkinsonism gene ATP13A2 causes neuronal ceroid-lipofuscinosis. Human Molecular Genetics, 2012; p. 1–5.

[151] Lill CM, et al. Comprehensive research synopsis and systematic meta-analyses in Parkinson's disease genetics: The PDGene database. PLoS Genet. 2012;8(3):e1002548. doi: 10.1371/journal.pgen.1002548. Epub 2012 Mar 15.

[152] Dai D, et al. Association of four GSTs gene polymorphisms with Parkinson disease: A meta-analysis. Advances in Bioscience and Biotechnology, 2014, 5; p. 100-107.

[153] Gencer M, et al. DNA Repair Genes in Parkinson's Disease. Genetic Testing and Molecular Biomarkers. 2012; 16(6); p. 504-507.

[154] Molochnikov L, et al. A molecular signature in blood identifies early Parkinson's disease. Molecular Neurodegeneration 2012, 7:26; p. 1-10.

[155] Dhillon VS, Fenech M. Mutations that affect mitochondrial functions and their association with neurodegenerative diseases. Mutation Research/Reviews in Mutation Research, 2014; Volume 759; p. 1–13.

[156] Desplats P, et al. Combined exposure to Maneb and Paraquat alters transcriptional regulation of neurogenesis-related genes in mice models of Parkinson's disease. Mol Neurodegener. 2012; 7: 49. Published online Sep 28, 2012. doi: 10.1186/1750-1326-7-49.

[157] Goldman SM, et al. Peptidoglycan Recognition Protein Genes and Risk of Parkinson's Disease. Movement Disorders, 2014; Vol. 29, No. 9; p. 1171-1180.

[158] Chen D, et al. Genetic analysis of the ATG7 gene promoter in sporadic Parkinson's disease. Neurosci Lett. 2013; 534; p. 193-198.

[159] Rhodes SL, et al. Pesticides that inhibit the ubiquitin–proteasome system: Effect measure modification by genetic variation in SKP1 in Parkinson's disease. Environmental Research, 2013; Volume 126; p. 1–8.

[160] Noyce AJ, et al. Meta-analysis of early nonmotor features and risk factors for Parkinson disease. Annals of Neurology, 2012; Volume 72, Issue 6; p. 893-901.

[161] Benito-Leon J, Louis ED, Bermejo-Pareja F. Risk of incident Parkinson's disease and parkinsonism in essential tremor: a population-based study. Journal of Neurology, Neurosurgery & Psychiatry 2009; Volume 80; p. 423-425.

[162] Nilsson FM, Kessing LV, Bolwig TG. Increased risk of developing Parkinson's disease for patients with major affective disorder: a register study. Acta Psychiatr Scand. 2001;104(5); p.380-386.

[163] Healy DG, et al. Tau gene and Parkinson's disease: a case–control study and meta-analysis. J Neurol Neurosurg Psychiatry 2004;75; p.962–965.

[164] Rosen AR, et al. Evidence of shared risk for Alzheimer's disease and Parkinson's disease using family history. Neurogenetics. 2007; 8(4): p. 263–270.

[165] Nalls MA, et al. Genetic comorbidities in Parkinson's disease. Hum. Mol. Genet., 2014; 23 (3); p. 831-841.

[166] Aden E, at al. Dietary intake and olfactory function in patients with newly diagnosed Parkinson's disease: a case-control study. Nutritional Neuroscience, 2011; Volume 14, Issue 1; p. 25-31.

[167] Isihura L, Brayne C, A Systematic review of nutritional risk factors of Parkinson's disease. Nutrition Research Reviews, 2005; 18; p.259-282.

[168] Roede JR, et al. Serum Metabolomics of Slow vs. Rapid Motor Progression Parkinson's Disease: a Pilot Study. PLOS ONE, 2013; Volume 8, Issue 10; e77629.

[169] Courtemanche C, et al, Folate deficiency and ionizing radiation cause DNA breaks in primary human lymphocytes: A comparison. FASEB J. 2004; 18; p. 2009-2011.

[170] Martin A, Joseph JA, Cuervo AM. Stimulatory effect of vitamin C on autophagy in glial cells. J Neurochem. 2002;82(3); p.538-549.

[171] Wu S, Sun J. Vitamin D, Vitamin D Receptor, and Macroautophagy in Inflammation and Infection. Discov Med. 2011; 11(59); p. 325–335.

[172] Martina JA, et al. The nutrient-responsive transcription factor TFE3 promotes autophagy, lysosomal biogenesis, and clearance of cellular debris. Sci Signal. 2014;7(309):ra9. doi: 10.1126/scisignal.2004754.

[173] Fernstrom JD. Effects on the diet on brain neurotransmitters. Metabolism. 1977;26(2); p.207-223.

[174] Odjakova M, Hadjiivanova C. Animal Neurotransmitter Substances in Plants. Bulg. J. Plant Physiol., 1997; 23(1–2) ;p. 94–102.

[175] Gao X, et al, Habitual intake of dietary flavonoids and risk of Parkinson disease. Neurology. 2012; 78(15); p.1138–1145.

[176] Mofort A, Wutz A. Breathing-in epigenetic change with vitamin C. EMBO reports, 2013; Vol. 14, No. 4; p.337-344.

[177] Iqbal K, Khan A, Khattak M. Biological significance of Ascorbic Acid (Vitamin C) on Human Health—A Review. Pakistan Journal of Nutrition., 2004; 3(1); p. 5-13.

[178] Urrutia P, et al. Inflammation alters the expression of DMT1, FPN1 and hepcidin, and it causes iron accumulation in central nervous system cells. Journal of Neurochemistry, 2013; Volume 126, Issue 4; p. 541–549.

[179] Qian L, Flood PM, Hong J, Neuroinflammation is a key player in Parkinson's disease and a prime target for therapy, Journal of Neural Transmission. 2010; 117(8); p. 971–979.

[180] Seidl S, Potashkin J. The Promise of Neuroprotective Agents in Parkinson's Disease. Front Neurol. 2011; 2: 68. doi: 10.3389/fneur.2011.00068

[181] Melnik BC. Milk—The promoter of chronic Western diseases. Medical Hypotheses, 2009; 72(6); p.631-639.

[182] Pérez-Revuelta BI, et al. Metformin lowers Ser-129 phosphorylated α-synuclein levels via mTOR-dependent protein phosphatase 2A activation. Cell Death Dis. 2014;5: e1209. doi: 10.1038/cddis.2014.175.

[183] Melnik BC. Dietary intervention in acne: Attenuation of increased mTORC1 signaling promoted by Western diet. Dermato-Endocrinology, 2012; 4:1; p. 20–32.

[184] Bolca S, van de Wiele T, Possemiers S. Gut metabotypes govern health effects of dietary polyphenols. Current Opinion in Biotechnology 2012; 24; p. 1-6.

[185] Li Z, et al. Essential roles of enteric neuronal serotonin in gastrointestinal motility and the development/survival of enteric dopaminergic neurons. J Neuroscience, 2011;31(24); p.8998-9009.

[186] Clairembault T, Leclair-Visonneau L, Neunlist M, Derkinderen P. Enteric glial cells: New players in Parkinson's disease? Mov Disord. 2014 Aug 7. doi: 10.1002/mds.25979.

[187] Devos D, et al. Colonic inflammation in Parkinson's disease. Neurobiol Dis., 2013;50; p.42-48.

[188] Geddes L. Switching diets transforms your gut bugs in 24 hours. New Scientist, 2013; Volume 220, Issue 2947; p. 11.

[189] Hsu TM, Kanoski SE. Blood-brain barrier disruption: mechanistic links between Western diet consumption and dementia. Front Aging Neurosci. 2014 May 9; 6:88. doi: 10.3389/fnagi.2014.00088.

[190] Wang YZ, Xu TL. Acidosis, Acid-Sensing Ion Channels, and Neuronal Cell Death. Mol Neurobiol, 2011;44 p.350–358.

[191] Silva BA, Breydo L, Uversky VN. Targeting the chameleon: a focused look at α-synuclein and its roles in neurodegeneration. Mol Neurobiol. 2013;47(2); p.446-459.

[192] Buel AK, et al. Solution conditions determine the relative importance of nucleation and growth processes in α-synuclein aggregation. PNAS, 2014; vol. 111, no. 21; p. 7671–7676.

[193] Pizzorno J, Frassetto LA, Katzinger J. Diet-induced acidosis: is it real and clinically relevant? Br J Nutr. 2010;103(8); p.1185-1194.

[194] Kreilaus F, Jenner AM. The effect of a western diet on the synthesis and metabolism of cholesterol in the brain. 33rd Meeting of the Australian Neuroscience Society: Program, Abstracts & List of Registrants, 2013, p. 124.

[195] Kummerow FA. The Cause for Heart Disease and Strokes. Journal of Nutritional Therapeutics, 2013; 2; p. 122-126.

[196] Tsai S, Liu W, Yin M. Trans Fatty Acids Enhanced Beta-Amyloid Induced Oxidative Stress in Nerve Growth Factor Differentiated PC12 Cells. Neurochemical Research, 2012; Volume 37, Issue 4; p 786-794.

[197] Gao X, et al. Prospective study of dietary pattern and risk of Parkinson disease. American Journal of Clinical Nutrition 2007;86; p. 1486 –1494.

[198] Rotermund C, et al. Diet-induced obesity accelerates the onset of terminal phenotypes in α-synuclein transgenic mice. Journal of Neurochemistry, 2014. DOI: 10.1111/jnc.12813

[199] Morris JK, Bomhoff GL, Stanford JA, Geiger PC. Neurodegeneration in an animal model of Parkinson's disease is exacerbated by a high-fat diet. Am J Physiol Regul Integr Comp Physiol 299, 2010; p. R1082–R1090.

[200] Choi JY, et al. Enhanced susceptibility to 1-methyl-4-phenyl-1,2,3,6-tetrahydropyridine neurotoxicity in high-fat diet-induced obesity. Free Radical Biology and Medicine, 2005; Volume 38, Issue 6; p. 806–816.

[201] Prior LJ, et al. Exposure to a High-Fat Diet Alters Leptin Sensitivity and Elevates Renal Sympathetic Nerve Activity and Arterial Pressure in Rabbits. Hypertension. 2010;55; p.862-868.

[202] Vucetic Z, Carlin JL, Totoki K, Reyes TM. Epigenetic dysregulation of the dopamine system in diet-induced obesity. Journal of Neurochemistry, 2012; 120; p. 891-898.

[203] Adeva MM, Souto G. Diet-induced metabolic acidosis. Clin Nutr. 2011;30(4); p.416-421.

[204] Singh R, Cuervo AM. Autophagy in the Cellular Energetic Balance. Cell Metabolism, 2011; 13; p. 495-504.

[205] Waller-Evans H, et al. Nutrigenomics of High Fat Diet Induced Obesity in Mice Suggests Relationships between Susceptibility to Fatty Liver Disease and the Proteasome. PLOS One, 2013; DOI: 10.1371/journal.pone.0082825

[206] Pistell PJ, et al. Cognitive Impairment Following High Fat Diet Consumption is Associated with Brain Inflammation. Journal of Neuroimmunology. 2010; 219(1-2): p. 25–32.

[207] Gutiérrez Ruiz MC, et al. High cholesterol diet modifies the repairing effect of the hepatocyte growth factor. Gac Med Mex., 2012;148(3); p.236-242.

[208] Kanoski SE, Zhang Y, Zheng W, Davidson TL. The Effects of a High-Energy Diet on Hippocampal Function and Blood-Brain Barrier Integrity in the Rat. Journal of Alzheimer's Disease, 2010; 21; p. 207–219.

[209] Poschmann G, et al. High-Fat Diet Induced Isoform Changes of the Parkinson's Disease Protein DJ-1. J. Proteome Res., 2014; 13(5); p. 2339–2351.

[210] Zondler L, et al. DJ-1 interactions with α-synuclein attenuate aggregation and cellular toxicity in models of Parkinson's disease. Cell Death Dis. 2014 Jul 24;5:e1350. doi: 10.1038/cddis.2014.307.

[211] Kim KY, et al. Parkin is a lipid-responsive regulator of fat uptake in mice and mutant human cells. J Clin Invest. 2011;121(9); p.3701–3712.

[212] Lingnert H, et al. Acrylamide in food: mechanisms of formation and influencing factors during heating of foods. Scandinavian Journal of Nutrition, 2002; 46 (4): p. 159–172.

[213] Luo J, Shi R. Acrolein induces oxidative stress in brain mitochondria. Neurochemistry International, 2005; 46; p. 243–252.

[214] Jeong MS, Kang JH. Acrolein, the toxic endogenous aldehyde, induces neurofilament-L aggregation. BMB reports, 2013, p. 635-639.

[215] http://www.atsdr.cdc.gov/toxprofiles/tp22-c1.pdf Accessed June 5, 2014.

[216] Walton JR. Functional impairment in aged rats chronically exposed to human range dietary aluminum equivalents. NeuroToxicology, 2009; Volume 30, Issue 2; p. 182–193.

[217] Francis H, Stevenson R. The longer-term impacts of Western diet on human cognition and the brain. Appetite, 2013; Volume 63, 1; p. 119–128.

[218] Simmonds SS, Lay J, Stocker SD. Dietary Salt Intake Exaggerates Sympathetic Reflexes and Increases Blood Pressure Variability in Normotensive Rats. HYPERTENSION AHA.114.03250. Published online before print June 9, 2014, doi: 10.1161/HYPERTENSIONAHA.114.03250.

[219] Liu YZ, et al. High-salt diet enhances hippocampal oxidative stress and cognitive impairment in mice. Neurobiology of Learning and Memory, 2014, Volume 114; p.10–15.

[220] Kleineweitfeld M, et al. Sodium chloride drives autoimmune disease by the induction of pathogenic T 17 cells. Nature, 2013; 496; p. 518–522.

[221] Hu WC. Parkinson disease is a TH17 dominant autoimmune disorder against accumulated alpha-synuclein. Quantitative Biology, 2013; arXiv:1403.3256 [q-bio. OT]

[222] Münch G, Westcott B, Menini T, Gugliucci A. Advanced glycation endproducts and their pathogenic roles in neurological disorders. Amino Acids, 2012;42(4); p.1221-1236.

[223] Lee D, Park CW, Paik SR, Choi KY. The modification of alpha-synuclein by dicarbonyl compounds inhibits its fibril-forming process. Biochim Biophys Acta., 2009;1794(3); p.421-430.

[224] Ankrah NA, Appiah-Opong R. Methylgloxal depletes glutathione. Toxicology Letters, 1999; Volume 109, Issues 1–2; p. 61–67.

[225] Tikellis C, et al. Cardiac inflammation associated with a Western diet is mediated via activation of RAGE by AGEs. Am J Physiol Endocrinol Metab, 2008; 295; p. E323–E330.

[226] Fang F, et al. RAGE-dependent signaling in microglia contributes to neuroinflammation, Abeta accumulation, and impaired learning/memory in a mouse model of Alzheimer's disease. FASEB J. 2010;24(4); p.1043-1055.

[227] Uribarri J, et al. Advanced Glycation End Products in Foods and a Practical Guide to Their Reduction in the Diet. J Am Diet Assoc., 2010; 110(6); p.911–916.

[228] Birlouez-Aragon I, et al. A diet based on high-heat-treated foods promotes risk factors for diabetes mellitus and cardiovascular diseases. Am J Clin Nutr., 2010; 91; p.1220–1226.

[229] Savica R, Grossardt BR, Bower JH, Ahlskog JE, Rocca WA. Risk factors for Parkinson's disease may differ in men and women: an exploratory study. Horm Behav. 2013; 63(2); p.308-314.

[230] Ayton S, Lei P. Nigral Iron Elevation Is an Invariable Feature of Parkinson's Disease and Is a Sufficient Cause of Neurodgeneration. Hindawi Publishing Corporation, BioMed Research International, Volume 2014, Article ID 581256, 9 pages.

[231] Sripetchwandee J, Pipatpiboon N, Chattipakorn N, Chattipakorn S. Combined Therapy of Iron Chelator and Antioxidant Completely Restores Brain Dysfunction Induced by Iron Toxicity. PLOS ONE, 2014; Volume 9, Issue 1; e85115; 15 pages.

[232] Zecca L, Youdim MBH, Riederer P, Connor JR. Iron, brain ageing and neurodegenerative disorders. Nature Reviews, 2004, Volume 5, p. 863-874.

[233] Powers KM, et al. Parkinson's disease risks associated with dietary iron, manganese, and other nutrient intakes. Neurology, 2003; vol. 60, no. 11; p. 1761-1766.

[234] Elseweidy MM, Abd El-Baky AE. Effect of dietary iron overload in rat brain: oxidative stress, neurotransmitter level and serum metal ion in relation to neurodegenerative disorders. Indian J Exp Biol. 2008;46(12); p.855-858.

[235] Geissler C, Singh M. Iron, Meat and Health. Nutrients 2011, 3(3); p. 283-316.

[236] Peng J, et al. Iron and Paraquat as Synergistic Environmental Risk Factors in Sporadic Parkinson's Disease Accelerate Age-Related Neurodegeneration. The Journal of Neuroscience, 2007; 27(26); p. 6914-6922.

[237] Du M, Shen QW, Zhu MJ, Ford SP. Leucine stimulates mammalian target of rapamycin signaling in C2C12 myoblasts in part through inhibition of adenosine monophosphate-activated protein kinase. J Anim Sci. 2007;85(4); p.919-927.

[238] Johnson CC, Gorell JM, Rybicki BA, Sanders K, Peterson EL. Adult nutrient intake as a risk factor for Parkinson's disease. International Journal of Epidemiology. 1999;28(6); p.1102-1109.

[239] http://www.usda.gov/oig/webdocs/24601-08-KC.pdf . Accessed August 3, 2013.

[240] Glaros TG, et al. Causes and consequences of low grade endotoxemia and inflammatory diseases . Frontiers in Bioscience 2013, 5; p. 754-765.

[241] Kuhn W, Müller T, Grosse H, Rommelspacher H. Elevated levels of harman and norharman in cerebrospinal fluid of parkinsonian patients. J Neural Transm. 1996;103(12); p.1435-1440.

[242] Louis ED, Zheng W. β-Carboline Alkaloids and Essential Tremor: Exploring the Environmental Determinants of One of the Most Prevalent Neurological Diseases. ScientificWorldJournal. ; 10: 1783–1794. doi:10.1100/tsw.2010.159.

[243] Oz F, Kaya M. The inhibitory effect of red pepper on heterocyclic aromatic amines in fried beef longissimus dorsi muscle. Journal of Food Processing and Preservation, 2011, Volume 35, Issue 6; p. 806–812.

[244] Oz F, Kaya M. The inhibitory effect of black pepper on formation of heterocyclic aromatic amines in high-fat meatball. Food Control, 2011, Volume 22, Issues 3–4; p. 596–600.

[245] Smith JS, Ameri F, Gadgil P. Effect of marinades on the formation of heterocyclic amines in grilled beef steaks. J Food Sci. 2008;73(6); p.T100-105.

[246] Jiang W, Ju C, Jiang H, Zhang D. Dairy foods intake and risk of Parkinson's disease: a dose-response meta-analysis of prospective cohort studies. Eur J Epidemiol. 2014 Jun 4. PMID: 24894826

[247] Chen H, et al, Consumption of Dairy Products and Risk of Parkinson's Disease. American Journal of Epidemiology, 2007; Vol. 165, No. 9; p.998-1006.

[248] Grant WB, The role of milk protein in increasing risk of Parkinson's disease. European Journal of Epidemiology, 2013, 28:357.

[249] Holt C, Carver JA. Darwinian transformation of a 'scarcely nutritious fluid' into milk. Journal of Evolutionary Biology, 2012; Volume 25, Issue 7; p. 1253–1263.

[250] Westermark P, Andersson A, Westermark GT. Islet Amyloid Polypeptide, Islet Amyloid, and Diabetes Mellitus. Physiological Reviews, 2011; Vol. 91,no. 3; p. 795-826.

[251] Thorn DC, et al. Amyloid fibril formation by bovine milk alpha s2-casein occurs under physiological conditions yet is prevented by its natural counterpart, alpha s1-casein. Biochemistry. 2008;47(12); p.3926-3936.

[252] Ostman EM, et al. Inconsistency between glycemic and insulinemic responses to regular and fermented milk products. Am J Clin Nutr., 2001;74; p. 96–100.

[253] Mansourbahmani M, et al. Study of Existing Radon In Milk and Its Effect on Body Organs. International Journal of Advanced Biological and Biomedical Research, 2013; Volume 1, Issue 8; p. 802-812.

[254] Nauta MJ, van der Giessen JW. Human exposure to Mycobacterium paratuberculosis via pasteurised milk: a modelling approach. Vet Rec., 1998;143(11); p.293-296.

[255] Dow CD. M. Paratuberculosis and Parkinson's Disease - Is this a Trigger. Medical Hypotheses, 2014. DOI: http://dx.doi.org/10.1016/j.mehy.2014.09.025

[256] Turnbaugh PJ. Microbiology: fat, bile and gut microbes. Nature, 012;487(7405); p.47-48.

[257] Baron EJ. Bilophila wadsworthia: a unique Gram-negative anaerobic rod. Anaerobe. 1997; 3(2-3); p.83-86.

[258] Adamidis D, et al. Fiber intake and childhood appendicitis. International Journal of Food Sciences and Nutrition, 2000; Vol. 51, No. 3; p. 153-157.

[259] Bollinger RR, et al. Biofilms in the large bowel suggest an apparent function of the human vermiform appendix. Journal of Theoretical Biology, 2007; Volume 249, Issue 4; p. 826–831.

[260] Gray MT, et al. Alpha-synuclein in the appendiceal mucosa of neurologically intact subjects. Movement Disorders, 2014; Volume 29, Issue 8; p. 991–998.

[261] Melnik BC, John SM, Schmitz G. Milk is not just food but most likely a genetic transfection system activating mTORC1 signaling for postnatal growth. Nutrition Journal 2013, 12:103.

[262] Jung CH, et al. mTOR regulation of autophagy. FEBS Lett. 2010;584(7); p.1287-1295.

[263] Yokel RA, Hicks CL, Florence RL. Aluminum bioavailability from basic sodium aluminum phosphate, an approved food additive emulsifying agent, incorporated in cheese. Food Chem Toxicol. 2008;46(6); p.2261-2266.

[264] Yokel RA. Aluminum in Food – The Nature and Contribution of Food Additives. In: Food Additive, edited by Yehia El-Samragy, ISBN 978-953-51-0067-6, 268 pages, Publisher: InTech.DOI: 10.5772/1521

[265] Saiyed SM, Yokel RA. Aluminium content of some foods and food products in the USA, with aluminium food additives. Food Additives & Contaminants, 2005; Volume 22, Issue 3; DOI:10.1080/02652030500073584

[266] Münch G, Westcott B, Menini T, Gugliucci A. Advanced glycation endproducts and their pathogenic roles in neurological disorders. Amino Acids, 2012;42(4); p.1221-1236.

[267] Horton L, et al. Comprehensive assessment of alcohol-related brain damage (ARBD): gap or chasm in the evidence? Journal of Psychiatric and Mental Health Nursing; article first published online:2014; DOI: 10.1111/jpm.12156

[268] Lippai D, et al. Alcohol-induced IL-1β in the brain is mediated by NLRP3/ASC inflammasome activation that amplifies neuroinflammation. Journal of Leukocyte Biology, 2013; vol. 94, no. 1; p. 171-182.

[269] Landau AM, Kouassi E, Siegrist-Johnstone R, Desbarats J. Proteasome inhibitor model of Parkinson's disease in mice is confounded by neurotoxicity of the ethanol vehicle. Mov Disord. 2007; 22(3); p.403-407.

[270] Volkow ND, et al. Decreases in Dopamine Receptors but not in Dopamine Transporters in Alcoholics. Alcoholism: Clinical and Experimental Research, 1996; Vol. 20, No. 9; p. 1594-1598.

[271] Zahr NM, Kaufman KL, Harper CG. Clinical and pathological features of alcohol-related brain damage. Nature Reviews Neurology 7, 284-294 (May 2011) | doi:10.1038/nrneurol.2011.42

[272] Bousquet-Dubouch MP, et al. Chronic ethanol feeding affects proteasome-interacting proteins. Proteomics. 2009; 9(13); p. 3609-3622.

[273] Kones R. Parkinson's Disease: Mitochondrial Molecular Pathology, Inflammation, Statins, and Therapeutic Neuroprotective Nutrition. Nutrition in Clinical Practice 2010 25: p. 371-389.

[274] Miyake Y, et al. Dietary fat intake and risk of Parkinson's disease: a case-control study in Japan. J Neurol Sci. 2010 Jan 15;288(1-2): p. 117-122.

[275] Cardoso HD, et al. Differential vulnerability of substantia nigra and corpus striatum to oxidative insult induced by reduced dietary levels of essential fatty acids. Front Hum Neurosci. 2012 Aug 30; 6:249. doi: 10.3389/fnhum.2012.00249. eCollection 2012.

[276] Simopoulos AP. The importance of the ratio of omega-6/omega 3 essential fatty acids. Biomedical Pharmacotherapy, 2002; 56 (8): p. 365-379.

[277] Yehuda S, "Omega-6/Omega-3 Ratio and Brain-Related Functions," in: Simopoulos AP, Cleland LG (editors): Omega-6/Omega-3 Essential fatty Acid Ratio: The Scientific Evidence. Basel, Karger, 2003; p. 37-56.

[278] Wood KE, et al. Incorporating macadamia oil and butter to reduce dietary omega-6 polyunsaturated fatty acid intake. Nutrition & Dietetics, 2013; Volume 70, Issue 2; p. 94–100.

[279] Aviles-Olmos I, Limousin P, Lees A, Foltynie T. Parkinson's disease, insulin resistance and novel agents of neuroprotection. Brain. 2013; 136(Pt 2); p.374-384.

[280] Zhao S, Zhang L, Xu Z, Chen W. Neurotoxic effects of iron overload under high glucose concentration. Neural Regeneration Research, 2013, Volume 8, Issue 36; p. 3423-3433.

[281] Hipkiss AR. Parkinson's Disease and Type-2 Diabetes: Methylglyoxal may be a Common Causal Agent; Carnosine
could be Protective. Mol Med Ther., 2012; 1:2; doi:10.4172/2324-8769.1000104

[282] Miranda HV, et al. Posttranslational modifcations of blood-derived alpha-synuclein as biochemical markers for Parkinson's disease. Scientific Reports, 2017, 7: 13713 | DOI:10.1038/s41598-017-14175-5

[283] Gatto NM, Cockburn M, Bronstein J, Manthripragada AD, Ritz B. Well-water consumption and Parkinson's disease in rural California. Environ Health Perspectives. 2009;117(12); p.1912-1918.

[284] Thiruchelvam M, et al. The Nigrostriatal Dopaminergic System as a Preferential Target of Repeated Exposures to Combined Paraquat and Maneb: Implications for Parkinson's Disease. The Journal of Neuroscience, 2000; 20(24): p. 9207-9214.

[285] Svendsen C, Ragas AMJ, Dorne JLCM. Contaminants in Organic and Conventional Food: The Missing Link Between Contaminant Levels and Health Effects, in: Health Benefits of Organic Food: Effects of the Environment, edited by D. Ian Givens, CABI, 2008, p. 121.

[286] Lu C, et al. Organic Diets Significantly Lower Children's Dietary Exposure to Organophosphorus Pesticides. Environmental Health Perspectives, Volume 114, Number 2, February 2006.

[287] http://www.epa.gov/oppfead1/international/trade/ Accessed August 31, 2013.

[288] Sharma S, Ebadi M. Metallothioneins as early and sensitive biomarkers of redox signaling in neurodegenerative disorders. IIOABJ, 2011, vol. 2, issue 6; p. 98-106.

[289] Baltaci AK, Mogulkuc R. Leptin and zinc relation: In regulation of food intake and immunity. Indian J Endocrinol Metab. 2012; 16(Suppl 3); p. S611–S616.

[290] Russo AJ. Decreased Serum Hepatocyte Growth Factor (HGF) in Individuals with Bipolar Disorder Normalizes after Zinc and Anti-oxidant Therapy. Nutr Metab Insights. 2010;3; p.49-55.

[291] Chondrogianni N, et al. Proteasome activation delays aging in vitro and in vivo. Free Radical Biology and Medicine, 2014; 71; p. 303-320.

[292] Miyakea Y, et al. Dietary intake of metals and risk of Parkinson's disease: A case-control study in Japan. Journal of the Neurological Sciences, 2011; Volume 306, Issues 1–2; p. 98–102.

[293] Pillai R, Uyehara-Lock JH, Bellinger FP. Selenium and selenoprotein function in brain disorders. IUBMB Life, 2014;66(4); p.229-239.

[294] González S. Serum selenium is associated with plasma homocysteine concentrations in elderly humans. J Nutr. 2004;134(7); p.1736-1740.

[295] Baker DH, Czarnecki-Maulden GL. Pharmacologic role of cysteine in ameliorating or exacerbating mineral toxicities. Journal of Nutrition 1987;117; p.1003–1110.

[296] Daubner SC, Le T, Wang S. Tyrosine Hydroxylase and Regulation of Dopamine Synthesis. Arch Biochem Biophys. 2011; 1; 508(1); p. 1–12.

[297] van der Hulst RR, von Meyenfeldt MF, Soeters PB. Glutamine: an essential amino acid for the gut. Nutrition, 1996;12(11-12 Suppl); p.S78-S81.

[298] Sakiyama T, et al. Glutamine increases autophagy under Basal and stressed conditions in intestinal epithelial cells. Gastroenterology, 2009; 136(3); p. 924-932.

[299] Hipkiss AR. Could carnosine or related structures suppress Alzheimer's disease? J Alzheimers Dis. 2007;11(2); p.229-240.

[300] Hipkiss AR, et al. Carnosine: can understanding its actions on energy metabolism and protein homeostasis inform its therapeutic potential? Chemistry Central Journal, 2013; 7:38; 9 pages.

[301] Stabler SP. Vitamin B12 Deficiency. New England Journal of Medicine, 2013; 368; 2; p. 149-160.

[302] Bousquet M, et al. Beneficial effects of dietary omega-3 polyunsaturated fatty acid on toxin-induced neuronal degeneration in an animal model of Parkinson's disease. The FASEB Journal, 2008; Vol. 22; p. 1213-1225.

[303] Kamel F, et al. Dietary fat intake, pesticide use, and Parkinson's disease. Parkinsonism & Related Disorders, 2014; Volume 20, Issue 1; p. 82–87.

[304] Calderón-Garcidueñas, L. et al. "Brain Inflammation and Alzheimer's-Like Pathology in Individuals Exposed to Severe Air Pollution." Toxicologic Pathology, 2004, 32 (6): p. 650–658.

[305] Turk HF, Chapkin RS. Membrane lipid raft organization is uniquely modified by n-3 polyunsaturated fatty acids. Prostaglandins, Leukotrienes and Essential Fatty Acids, 2013, Volume 88, Issue 1; p. 43-47.

[306] Fabelo N, et al. Severe Alterations in Lipid Composition of Frontal Cortex Lipid Rafts from Parkinson's Disease and Incidental Parkinson's Disease. Molecular Medicine 17, 2011; (9-10); p. 1107-1118.

[307] Hatano T, et al. Leucine-rich repeat kinase 2 associates with lipid rafts. Human Molecular Genetics, Volume 16, Issue 6; p. 678-690.

[308] Fabelo N, et al. Severe Alterations in Lipid Composition of Frontal Cortex Lipid Rafts from Parkinson's Disease and Incidental Parkinson's Disease. Mol Med. 2011;17(9-10); p.1107-1118.

[309] Zimmer L, Delpal S, Guilloteau D, Aïoun J, Durand G, Chalon S. Chronic n-3 polyunsaturated fatty acid deficiency alters dopamine vesicle density in the rat frontal cortex. Neurosci Lett. 2000;284(1-2):25-28.

[310] Tanriover G, et al. The effects of docosahexaenoic acid on glial derived neurotrophic factor and neurturin in bilateral rat model of Parkinson's disease. Folia Histochem Cytobiol. 2010;48(3): p. 434-441.

[311] Calder PC. Omega-3 Fatty Acids and Inflammatory Processes. Nutrients, 2010; 2; p. 355-374.

[312] Luyer MDP, Habes Q, van Hak R, Buurman W. Nutritional stimulation of the autonomic nervous system. World J Gastroenterol 2011; 17(34); p. 3859-3863.

[313] Pifferi F, et al. n-3 Fatty acids modulate brain glucose transport in endothelial cells of the blood-brain barrier. Prostaglandins Leukot Essent Fatty Acids. 2007;77(5-6); p. 279-286.

[314] Mazza M, et al. Omega-3 fatty acids and antioxidants in neurological and psychiatric diseases: An overview. Progress in Neuro-Psychopharmacology and Biological Psychiatry, 2007; Volume 31, Issue 1; p. 12–26.

[315] http://www.nrdc.org/health/effects/mercury/guide.asp Accessed November 21, 2013.

[316] Lu Z, et al. An Evaluation of the Vitamin D3 Content in Fish: Is the Vitamin D Content Adequate to Satisfy the Dietary Requirement for Vitamin D? J Steroid Biochem Mol Biol. ,2007;103(3-5); p.642–644.

[317] Andersson U, Tracey KJ. Neural reflexes in inflammation and immunity. J. Exp. Med., 2012; Vol. 209, No. 6; p. 1057-1068.

[318] Friedrichs W, Ruparel SB, Marciniak RA, deGraffenried L. Omega-3 fatty acid inhibition of prostate cancer progression to hormone independence is associated with suppression of mTOR signaling and androgen receptor expression. Nutr Cancer. 2011;63(5); p.771-777.

[319] http://www.nrdc.org/health/effects/mercury/guide.asp Accessed November 21, 2013.

[320] Siscar R, Koenig S, Torreblanca A, Solé M. The role of metallothionein and selenium in metal detoxification in the liver of deep-sea fish from the NW Mediterranean Sea. Sci Total Environ., 2014;466-467; p.898-905.

[321] Nesheim MC, Nestle M. Advice for fish consumption: challenging dilemmas. American Journal of Clinical Nutrition 2014;99; p.973-974.

[322] Fall PA, Fredrikson M, Axelson O, Granerus AK. Nutritional and occupational factors influencing the risk of Parkinson's disease: A case-control study in southeastern Sweden. Movement Disorders, 1999, 14; p. 28–37.

[323] Wurtman RJ, Fernstrom JD. Control of brain monoamine synthesis by diet and plasma amino acids. Am J Clin Nutr, 1975; Vol. 28, No. 6; p. 638-647.

[324] Niculescu MD, Zeisel SH. Diet, methyl donors and DNA methylation: interactions between dietary folate, methionine and choline. J Nutr. 2002;132(8 Suppl); p.2333S-2335S.

[325] Pallauf K, Giller K, Huebbe P, Rimbach G. Nutrition and Healthy Ageing: Calorie Restriction or Polyphenol-Rich "MediterrAsian" Diet? Oxidative Medicine and Cellular Longevity, Volume 2013, Article ID 707421, 14 pages.

[326] Iriti M, Vitalini S, Fico G, Faoro F. Neuroprotective Herbs and Foods from Different Traditional Medicines and Diets. Molecules, 2010, 15; p. 3517-3555.

[327] Camargo A, et al. Expression of proinflammatory, proatherogenic genes is reduced by the Mediterranean diet in elderly people. British Journal of Nutrition, 2012; Volume 108, Issue 03; p. 500-508.

[328] Okubo, H, et al. Dietary patterns and risk of Parkinson's disease: a case–control study in Japan. European Journal of Neurology, 2012; Volume 19, Issue 5; p. 681–688.

[329] Valente T, et al. A Diet Enriched in Polyphenols and Polyunsaturated Fatty Acids, LMN Diet, Induces Neurogenesis in the Subventricular Zone and Hippocampus of Adult Mouse Brain. Journal of Alzheimer's Disease, 2009; Volume 18, Number 4; p. 849-865.

[330] Alcalay RN, et al. The Association between Mediterranean Diet Adherence and Parkinson's Disease. Movement Disorders, 2012; Vol. 27, No. 6; p. 771-774.

[331] Lundberg JO, Carlstrom M, Larsen FJ, Weitzberg E. Roles of dietary inorganic nitrate in cardiovascular health and disease. Cardiovascular Research, 2011; 89; p. 525-532.

[332] Wong KH, Cheung PCK. Nutritional evaluation of some subtropical red and green seaweeds: Part I — proximate composition, amino acid profiles and some physico-chemical properties. Food Chemistry, 2000; Volume 71, Issue 4; p. 475–482.

[333] Shaltiel-Karyo R, et al. A Blood-Brain Barrier (BBB) Disrupter Is Also a Potent α-Synuclein (α-syn) Aggregation Inhibitor: A Novel Dual Mechanism of Mannitol

for the Treatment of Parkinson's Disease. J Biol Chem., 2013; 288(24); p.17579–17588.

[334] Fukuta K, Nakamura T. Induction of hepatocyte growth factor by fucoidan and fucoidan-derived oligosaccharides. J Pharm Pharmacol. 2008;60(4); p.499-503.

[335] Ma Y, et al. Association between dietary fiber and serum C-reactive protein. American Journal of Clinical Nutrition, 2006;83; p. 760–766.

[336] Huuskonen J, Suuronen T, Nuutinen T, Kyrylenko S, Salminen A. Regulation of microglial inflammatory response by sodium butyrate and short chain fatty acids. British Journal of Pharmacology, 2004; 141(5); p. 874–880.

[337] Anastasovska J, et al. Fermentable Carbohydrate Alters Hypothalamic Neuronal activity and Protects against the Obesogenic Environment.Nature, 2012; Vol. 20, No. 5; p. 1016-1023.

[338] Schrezenmeir J, de Vrese M. Probiotics, prebiotics, and synbiotics—approaching a definition. Am J Clin Nutr. 2001;73(2 Suppl); p.361S-364S.

[339] Moshfegh AJ, Friday JE, Goldman JP, Ahuja JK. Presence of inulin and oligofructose in the diets of Americans. J Nutr. 1999 Jul;129(7 Suppl):1407S-1411S.

[340] Kumazawa T, et al. Levels of pyrroloquinoline quinone in various foods. Biochem. J., 1995;307; p. 331-333.

[341] Panesar PS. Fermented Dairy Products: Starter Cultures and Potential Nutritional Benefits Food and Nutrition Sciences, 2011; 2; p. 47-51.

[342] Veiga P, et al. Changes of the human gut microbiome induced by a fermented milk product. Scientific Reports 4, Article number: 6328 doi:10.1038/srep06328.

[343] Nase L, et al. Effect of Long–Term Consumption of a Probiotic Bacterium, *Lactobacillus rhamnosus GG*, in Milk on Dental Caries and Caries Risk in Children. Caries Res., 2001;35; p.412–420.

[344] Oli MW, et al. Functional amyloid formation by *Streptococcus mutans*. Microbiology, 2012; 158; p. 2903-2916.

[345] Stilling RM, Dinan TG, Cryan JF. Microbial genes, brain & behaviour - epigenetic regulation of the gut-brain axis. Genes Brain Behav. 2014;13(1); p.69-86.

[346] Mengheri E. Health, Probiotics, and Inflammation. J Clin Gastroenterol, 2008; Volume 42, Supp. 3, Part 2; S177-S178.

[347] Valentini L, et al. Impact of personalized diet and probiotic supplementation on inflammation, nutritional parameters and intestinal microbiota— The "RISTOMED project": Randomized controlled trial in healthy older People. Clinical Nutrition, 2014; DOI: http://dx.doi.org/10.1016/j.clnu.2014.09.023

[348] Distruti E, et al. Modulation of Intestinal Microbiota by the Probiotic VSL#3 Resets Brain Gene Expression and Ameliorates the Age-Related Deficit in LTP. PLOS ONE, 2014; Volume 9, Issue 9; e106503; 11 pages.

349 Tillisch K, et al. Consumption of Fermented Milk Product With Probiotic Modulates Brain Activity. Gastroenterology. 2013;144(7); doi:10.1053/j.gastro.2013.02.043.

350 Kiyatkin EA, Sharma HS. Permeability of the blood-brain barrier depends on brain temperature. Neuroscience, 2009; 161(3); p. 926–939.

351 Ueki A, Otsuka M. Life style risks of Parkinson's disease: Association between decreased water intake and constipation. Journal of Neurology, 2004; Volume 251, Issue 7 Supplement; p. vii18-vii23.

352 Arnaud MJ. Mild dehydration: a risk factor of constipation? European Journal of Clinical Nutrition, 2003; 57, Suppl 2; p.S88–S95.

353 Lin CH, et al. Risk of Parkinson's disease following severe constipation: A nationwide population-based cohort study. Parkinsonism & Related Disorders, 2014; DOI: 10.1016/j.parkreldis.2014.09.026

354 Natale G, et al. Transmission of prions within the gut and toward the central nervous system. Prion, 2011; 5:3; p.142-149.

355 Kleiner SM. Water: An Essential But Overlooked Nutrient. Journal of the American Dietetic Association, 1999; Volume 99, Issue 2; p. 200–206.

356 https://www2.ca.uky.edu/enri/pubs/enri129.pdf Accessed November 29, 2014.

357 Depeint F, et al. Mitochondrial function and toxicity: role of the B vitamin family on mitochondrial energy metabolism. Chem Biol Interact, 27; 163 (1-2); p. 94-112.

358 Esteves AR, et al. Mitochondrial Dysfunction: The Road to Alpha-Synuclein Oligomerization in PD. Parkinson's Disease, Volume 2011, Article ID 693761, 20 pages; doi:10.4061/2011/693761.

359 Tufi R, et al. Enhancing nucleotide metabolism protects against mitochondrial dysfunction and neurodegeneration in a PINK1 model of Parkinson's disease. Nat Cell Biol., 2014;16(2); p.157–166.

360 Zhou M, et al. Neuronal death induced by misfolded prion protein is due to NAD+ depletion and can be relieved in vitro and in vivo by NAD+ replenishment. Brain, 2015; DOI: http://dx.doi.org/10.1093/brain/awv002

361 Murakami K, et al. Dietary intake of folate, vitamin B6, vitamin B12 and riboflavin and risk of Parkinson's disease: a case–control study in Japan. British Journal of Nutrition, 2010; Volume 104, Issue 05; p. 757-764.

362 Kamath, AF, et al. Elevated levels of homocysteine compromise blood-brain barrier integrity in mice. Blood, Vol. 107 No. 2, January 15, 2006, p. 591-593.

363 Zoccolella S, et al, Elevated Homocysteine Levels in Parkinson's Disease: Is there Anything Besides L-Dopa Treatment? Current Medicinal Chemistry, 2010; Volume 17, Number 3; p. 213-222.

[364] Werstuck GH, et al. Homocysteine-induced endoplasmic reticulum stress causes dysregulation of the cholesterol and triglyceride biosynthetic pathways. The Journal of Clinical Investigation, 2001; Volume 107, Number 10; p. 1263-1273.

[365] Duan W, et al. Dietary folate deficiency and elevated homocysteine levels endanger dopaminergic neurons in models of Parkinson's disease. Journal of Neurochemistry, 2002; Volume 80, Issue 1; p. 101–110.

[366] Handy DE, Zhang Y, Loscalzo J. Homocysteine down-regulates cellular glutathione peroxidase (GPx1) by decreasing translation. J Biol Chem. 2005;280(16); p. 15518-15525.

[367] McKillop DJ, et al. The effect of different cooking methods on folate retention in various foods that are amongst the major contributors to folate intake in the UK diet. Br J Nutr., 2002;88(6); p.681-688.

[368] Martignonia E, et al. Homocysteine and Parkinson's disease: A dangerous liaison? Journal of the Neurological Sciences, 2007; Volume 257, Issues 1–2; p.31–37.

[369] Huerta JM, et al. Folate and cobalamin synergistically decrease the risk of high plasma homocysteine in a nonsupplemented elderly institutionalized population. Clin Biochem., 2004;37(10); p.904-910.

[370] Huang LZ, et al. Nicotine is neuroprotective when administered before but not after nigrostriatal damage in rats and monkeys. Journal of Neurochemistry, 2009, Vol. 109; p. 826-837.

[371] Miksys S, Tyndale RF. Nicotine induces brain CYP enzymes: relevance to Parkinson's disease. Journal of Neural Transmission, 2006; Supplementa Volume 70; p. 177-180.

[372] Singh S, et al. Nicotine and caffeine-mediated modulation in the expression of toxicant responsive genes and vesicular monoamine transporter-2 in 1-methyl 4-phenyl-1,2,3,6-tetrahydropyridine-induced Parkinson's disease phenotype in mouse. Brain Research, 2008; Volume 1207; p. 193–206.

[373] Sheen SJ. Detection of Nicotine in Foods and Plant Materials. Journal of Food Science, 1988, 53; p. 1572–1573.

[374] Domino EF, Hornbach E, Demana T. The Nicotine Content of Common Vegetables. New England Journal of Medicine 1993; 329. P.437.

[375] Nielsen SS, et al. Nicotine from Edible Solanaceae and Risk of Parkinson Disease. Annals of Neurology, 2013; Volume 74; p. 472-477.

[376] Bjelakovic G, et al. Mortality in Randomized Trials of Antioxidant Supplements for Primary and Secondary Prevention. JAMA, 2007; Vol 297, No. 8; p. 842-857.

[377] Rietjens IM, et al. The pro-oxidant chemistry of the natural antioxidants vitamin C, vitamin E, carotenoids and flavonoids. Environ Toxicol Pharmacol., 2002; 11(3-4); p.321-333.

[378] Johnson WM, Wilson-Delfosse AL, Mieyal JJ. Dysregulation of Glutathione Homeostasis in Neurodegenerative Diseases. Nutrients, 2012; 4; p. 1399-1440.

[379] Currais A, Maher P. Functional Consequences of Age-Dependent Changes in Glutathione Status in the Brain. Antioxidants & Redox Signaling, 2013; 19(8); p.813-822.

[380] Li W, Busu C, Circu M, Aw TY. Glutathione in Cerebral Microvascular Endothelial Biology and Pathobiology: Implications for Brain Homeostasis. International Journal of Cell Biology, Volume 2012, Article ID 434971; p. 1-14.

[381] Johnson WM, Wilson-Delfosse AL, Mieyal JJ. Dysregulation of Glutathione Homeostasis in Neurodegenerative Diseases. Nutrients, 2012; 4; p. 1399-1440.

[382] Ribas V, Garcia-Ruiz C, Fernandez-Checa JC. Glutathione and mitochondria. Frontiers in Pharmacology, 2014, Vol. 5, Article 151; p. 1-19.

[383] Zeevalk GD, Razmpour R, Bernard LP. Glutathione and Parkinson's disease: is this the elephant in the room? Biomed Pharmacotherapy, 2008; 62(4); p. 236-49.

[384] Sian J, et al. Alteration in glutathione levels in Parkinson's disease and other neurodegenerative disorders affecting basal ganglia. Annals of Neurology, 1994; Volume 36, Issue 3; p. 348-355.

[385] Kaur D, Lee D, Ragapdan S, Andersen JK. Glutathione depletion in immortalized midbrain-derived dopaminergic neurons results in increases in the labile iron pool: Implications for Parkinson's disease. Free Radicals in Biology and Medicine, 2009; 46(5); p. 593-598.

[386] Jefferies H, et al. The Role of Glutathione in Intestinal Dysfunction. Journal of Investigative Surgery, 2003; Vol. 16, No. 6; p. 315-323.

[387] Vilar R, et al. Association of A313 G polymorphism (GSTP1*B) in the glutathione-S-transferase P1 gene with sporadic Parkinson's disease. European Journal of Neurology, 2007; 14; p. 156–161.

[388] Menegon A, et al. Parkinson's disease, pesticides, and glutathione transferase polymorphisms. The Lancet, Volume 352, Issue 9137, 24 October 1998; p. 1344–1346.

[389] Chen J. et al. GST P1, a novel downstream regulator of LRRK2, G2019S-induced neuronal cell death. Frontiers in Bioscience (Elite Ed). 2012; 4; p. 2365-77.

[390] Kang MJ, Gil SJ, Koh HC. Paraquat induces alternation of the dopamine catabolic pathways and glutathione levels in the substantia nigra of mice. Toxicology Letters, 2009; Volume 188, Issue 2; p. 148–152.

[391] Sheng J, Wu LG. Cysteine string protein α: a new role in vesicle recycling. Neuron, 2012;74(1); p. 6–8.

[392] Park Y, et al. Sulfur amino acid-free diet results in increased glutamate in human midbrain: A pilot magnetic resonance spectroscopy study. Nutrition, 2012; 28(3); p. 235–241.

[393] Ingenbleek Y, McCully KS. Vegetarianism produces subclinical malnutrition, hyperhomocysteinemia and atherogenesis. Nutrition, 2012; 28(2); p. 148-153.

[394] Sekhar RV, et al. Deficient synthesis of glutathione underlies oxidative stress in aging and can be corrected by dietary cysteine and glycine supplementation. American Journal of Clinical Nutrition, 2011; 94; p. 847–853.

[395] DeVera M, et al. Gout and the risk of Parkinson's disease: a cohort study. Arthritis Rheum. ,2008;59(11); p. 1549-1554.

[396] Gao X, et al. Diet, Urate, and Parkinson's Disease Risk in Men. American Journal of Epidemiology, 2008, Vol. 167, No. 7; p. 831-838.

[397] Bowman GL, et al. Uric Acid as a CNS Antioxidant. Journal of Alzheimers Disease, 2010; 19(4); p.1331–1336.

[398] Yamamoto T, et al. Effect of beer on the plasma concentrations of uridine and purine bases. Metabolism-Clinical and Experimental, 2002; Volume 51, Issue 10; p. 1317-1323.

[399] Cansev M, et al. Restorative Effects of Uridine Plus Docosahexaenoic Acid in a Rat Model of Parkinson's Disease. Neurosci Res. 2008; 62(3); p. 206–209.

[400] Foster DA. Reduced mortality and moderate alcohol consumption: The phospholipase D-mTOR connection. Cell Cycle. 2010; 9(7); p. 1291–1294.

[401] Zhang, D., Jiang, H. and Xie, J. Alcohol intake and risk of Parkinson's disease: A meta-analysis of observational studies. Mov. Disord. 2014; 29; p. 819–822.

[402] Yao J, et al. Xanthohumol, a Polyphenol Chalcone Present in Hops, Activating Nrf2 Enzymes To Confer Protection against Oxidative Damage in PC12 Cells. J. Agric. Food Chem., 2015; 63 (5); p. 1521–1531.

[403] Liu R, et al. Alcohol Consumption, Types of Alcohol, and Parkinson's Disease. PLOS ONE, 2013; Vol. 8; Issue 6; e66452.

[404] Gao M, et al. Habitual intake of dietary flavonoids and risk of Parkinson disease. Neurology 2012; 78; p.1138-1145.

[405] Huang WW, et al. Kaempferol induces autophagy through AMPK and AKT signaling molecules and causes G2/M arrest via downregulation of CDK1/cyclin B in SK-HEP-1 human hepatic cancer cells. Int J Oncol., 2013; 42(6); p.2069-2077.

[406] Kukull WA. An apple a day to prevent Parkinson disease. Neurology 2012; 78; p. 1112-1113.

[407] Davis JM, Murphy EA, Carmichael MD, Davis B. Quercetin increases brain and muscle mitochondrial biogenesis and exercise tolerance. Am J Physiol Regul Integr Comp Physiol, 2009, 296: R1071–R1077.

[408] Belinha I, et al. Quercetin Increases Oxidative Stress Resistance and Longevity in Saccharomyces cerevisiae. J. Agric. Food Chem., 2007; 55 (6) p.2446–2451.

[409] Chang HC, Yang YR, Wang PS, Wang RY. Quercetin Enhances Exercise-Mediated Neuroprotective Effects in Brain Ischemic Rats. Med Sci Sports Exerc. 2014 Feb 19. [Epub ahead of print]

[410] Pallauf K, Rimbach G. Autophagy, polyphenols and healthy ageing. Ageing Research Reviews, 2013; Volume 12, Issue 1; p. 237–252.

[411] Piperi C, Adamopoulos C, Dalagiorgou G, Diamanti-Kandarakis E, Papavassiliou AG. Crosstalk between advanced glycation and endoplasmic reticulum stress: emerging therapeutic targeting for metabolic diseases. J Clin Endocrinol Metab., 2012;97(7); p.2231-2242.

[412] Senadheera SP, Ekanayake S, Wanigatunge C. Antioxidant potential of green leafy porridges. Ceylon Med J. 2014; 59(1); p.4-8.

[413] Krishnamurthy S, Garabadu D, Reddy NR. Asparagus racemosus modulates the hypothalamic-pituitary-adrenal axis and brain monoaminergic systems in rats. Nutr Neurosci. 2013;16(6); p.255-261.

[414] Sanae M, Yasuo A. Green asparagus (Asparagus officinalis) prevented hypertension by an inhibitory effect on angiotensin-converting enzyme activity in the kidney of spontaneously hypertensive rats. J Agric Food Chem. 2013;61(23); p.5520-5525.

[415] Saxena G, et al. Neuroprotective effects of Asparagus Racemosus Linn root extract: An experimental and clinical evidence. Annals of Neurosciences, 2007; Volume 14, Issue 3.

[416] Zeisel SH. Is there a new component of the Mediterranean diet that reduces inflammation? Am J Clin Nutr., 2008; 87; p.277–278.

[417] Dirscherl K, et al. Luteolin triggers global changes in the microglial transcriptome leading to a unique anti-inflammatory and neuroprotective phenotype. J Neuroinflammation, 2010;7:3. doi: 10.1186/1742-2094-7-3.

[418] Ahmed JK, Salih HAM, Hadi AG. Anthocyanins in Red Beet Juice Act as Scavengers for Heavy Metals Ions such as Lead and Cadmium. International Journal of Science and Technology, 2013; Volume 2, No. 3; p. 269-274.

[419] Presley TD, et al. Acute effect of a high nitrate diet on brain perfusion in older adults. Nitric Oxide, 2011;24(1); p.34–42.

[420] McGuire SO, et al. Dietary supplementation with blueberry extract improves survival of transplanted dopamine neurons. Nutr. Neuroscience, 2006, 9; p. 251-258.

[421] Lau, FC, et al. J. Inhibitory effects of blueberry extract on the production of inflammatory mediators in lipopolysaccharide-activated BV2 microglia. Neuroscience Research., 2007, 85; p.1010-1017.

[422] Joseph JJ, et al. Reversals of Age-Related Declines in Neuronal Signal Transduction, Cognitive, and Motor Behavioral Deficits with Blueberry, Spinach, or Strawberry Dietary Supplementation. The Journal of Neuroscience, 15 September 1999, 19(18); p. 8114-8121.

[423] Patel MY, Panchal HV, Ghribi O, Benzeroual KE. The neuroprotective effect of fisetin in the MPTP model of Parkinson's disease. J Parkinsons Dis. 2012;2(4); p.287-302.

[424] Adhami VM, Syed DN, Khan N, Mukhtar H. Dietary flavonoid fisetin: a novel dual inhibitor of PI3K/Akt and mTOR for prostate cancer management. Biochem Pharmacol. 2012 November 15; 84(10): doi: 10.1016/j.bcp.2012.07.012.

[425] Tarozzi A, et al. Sulforaphane as a Potential Protective Phytochemical against Neurodegenerative Diseases. Oxidative Medicine and Cellular Longevity, Volume 2013, Article ID 415078, 10 pages.

[426] Dashwood RH, Ho E. Dietary histone deacetylase inhibitors: From cells to mice to man. Semin Cancer Biol., 2007; 17(5); p. 363–369.

[427] Lee JH, Jeong JK, Park SY. Sulforaphane-induced autophagy flux prevents prion protein-mediated neurotoxicity through AMPK pathway. Neuroscience, 2014;278; p.31-39.

[428] Rosen EM, et al. DIM (3,3'-diindolylmethane) confers protection against ionizing radiation by a unique mechanism. PNAS, October 14, 2013, doi: 10.1073/pnas.1308206110.

[429] Kong D, et al. Mammalian target of rapamycin repression by 3,3'-diindolylmethane inhibits invasion and angiogenesis in platelet-derived growth factor-D-over-expressing PC3 cells. Cancer Res. 2008; 68(6); p.1927-1934.

[430] Tilg H. Diet and intestinal immunity. N Engl J Med. 2012;366(2); p.181-183.

[431] Howatson G, et al. Effect of tart cherry juice (Prunus cerasus) on melatonin levels and enhanced sleep quality. European Journal of Nutrition, 2012; Volume 51, Issue 8; p. 909-916.

[432] Panickar AS, Polansky MM, Anderson RA. Cinnamon polyphenols attenuate cell swelling and mitochondrial dysfunction following oxygen-glucose deprivation in glial cells. Experimental Neurology 216 (2009); p. 420–427.

[433] Shaltiel-Karyo R, et al. Differential inhibition of α-synuclein oligomeric and fibrillar assembly in parkinson's disease model by cinnamon extract. Biochimica et Biophysica Acta (BBA) - General Subjects, 2012; Volume 1820, Issue 10; p. 1628–1635.

[434] Canet-Aviles RM, et al. The Parkinson's disease protein DJ-1 is neuroprotective due to cysteine-sulfinic acid-driven mitochondrial localization; Proc Natl Acad Sci U S A., 2004; 101(24); p. 9103–9108.

[435] Khasnavis S, Kalipada Pahan K. Sodium Benzoate, a Metabolite of Cinnamon and a Food Additive, Upregulates Neuroprotective Parkinson Disease Protein DJ-1 in Astrocytes and Neurons. J Neuroimmune Pharmacol. 2012; 7(2): p. 424–435.

[436] Jana A, et al. Up-Regulation of Neurotrophic Factors by Cinnamon and its Metabolite Sodium Benzoate: Therapeutic Implications for Neurodegenerative Disorders. Journal of Neuroimmune Pharmacology, 2013, Volume 8, Issue 3; p. 739-755.

[437] Adisakwattana S, et al. Cinnamic Acid and Its Derivatives Inhibit Fructose-Mediated Protein Glycation. Int. J. Mol. Sci., 2012; 13; p. 1778-1789.

[438] Hamza TH, et al. Genome-wide gene-environment study identifies glutamate receptor gene GRIN2A as a Parkinson's disease modifier gene via interaction with coffee. PLoS Genet. 2011;7(8):e1002237. doi: 10.1371/journal.pgen.1002237

[439] Aoyama K, et al. Caffeine and uric acid mediate glutathione synthesis for neuroprotection. Neuroscience, 2011; Volume 181; p. 206–215.

[440] Chen X, et al. Caffeine protects against MPTP-induced blood-brain barrier dysfunction in mouse striatum. Journal of Neurochemistry, 2008; Volume 107, Issue 4; p. 1147-1157.

[441] Chen X, et al. Caffeine blocks disruption of blood brain barrier in a rabbit model of Alzheimer's disease. Journal of Neuroinflammation 2008, 5:12 doi:10.1186/1742-2094-5-12.

[442] Brothers HM, Marchalant Y, Wenk G. Caffeine attenuates lipopolysaccharide-induced neuroinflammation. Neurosci Lett., 2010; 480(2); p. 97–100.

[443] Zhou H, Luo Y, Huang S. Updates of mTOR inhibitors. Anticancer Agents Med Chem, 2010; 10(7); p. 571-581.

[444] Saiki S, et al. Caffeine induces apoptosis by enhancement of autophagy via PI3K/Akt/mTOR/p70S6K inhibition. Autophagy, 2011;7(2); p.176-187.

[445] Singh S, et al. Nicotine and caffeine-mediated modulation in the expression of toxicant responsive genes and vesicular monoamine transporter-2 in 1-methyl 4-phenyl-1,2,3,6-tetrahydropyridine-induced Parkinson's disease phenotype in mouse. Brain Research, 2008; Volume 1207; p. 193–206.

[446] Piperi C, Adamopoulos C, Dalagiorgou G, Diamanti-Kandarakis E, Papavassiliou AG. Crosstalk between advanced glycation and endoplasmic reticulum stress: emerging therapeutic targeting for metabolic diseases. J Clin Endocrinol Metab., 2012;97(7); p.2231-2242.

[447] Mythri B, Srinvas M, Bharath M. Curcumin: A Potential Neuroprotective Agent in Parkinson's Disease. Current Pharmaceutical Design, 2012; Volume 18, Number 1; p. 91-99.

[448] Dashwood RH, Ho E. Dietary histone deacetylase inhibitors: From cells to mice to man. Semin Cancer Biol. 2007; 17(5); p. 363–369.

[449] Maiti P, Manna J, Veleri S, Frautschy S. Molecular Chaperone Dysfunction in Neurodegenerative Diseases and Effects of Curcumin. BioMed Research International, 2014; Article ID 495091, 14 pages

[450] Ahmad B, Lapidus LJ. Curcumin Prevents Aggregation in alpha-synuclein by Increasing the Reconfiguration Rate. The Journal of Biological Chemistry, 2012; 287; p. 9193-9199.

[451] Canfrán-Duque A, et al. Curcumin promotes exosomes/microvesicles secretion that attenuates lysosomal cholesterol traffic impairment. Mol Nutr Food Res., 2014; 58(4); p.687-697.

[452] Gomez-Pinilla F, Gomez A. The influence of Dietary Factors in Central Nervous System Plasticity and Injury Recovery. Physical Medicine and Rehabilitation 2011, Volume 3, p. S111-116.

[453] Ibid.

[454] Zhou H, Luo Y, Huang S. Updates of mTOR inhibitors. Anticancer Agents Med Chem, 2010; 10(7); p. 571-581.

[455] Anand P, et al. Biological activities of curcumin and its analogues (Congeners) made by man and Mother Nature. Biochemical Pharmacology; 2008; 76; p. 1590–1611.

[456] Baum L, Ng A. Curcumin interaction with copper and iron suggests one possible mechanism of action in Alzheimer's disease animal models. Journal of Alzheimer's Disease, 2004; 6; p. 367–377.

[457] Kelsey NA, Wilkins HM, Linseman DA. Nutraceutical Antioxidants as Novel Neuroprotective Agents. Molecules. 2010; 3;15(11); p. 7792-7814.

[458] Rabinkov A, et al. S-Allylmercaptoglutathione: the reaction product of allicin with glutathione possesses SH-modifying and antioxidant properties. Biochimica et Biophysica Acta (BBA) - Molecular Cell Research, 2000; Volume 1499, Issues 1–2; p. 144–153.

[459] Takechi R, et al. Nutraceutical agents with anti-inflammatory properties prevent dietary saturated-fat induced disturbances in blood–brain barrier function in wild-type mice. Journal of Neuroinflammation, 2013; 10:73; p. 1-12.

[460] Kannappan R, et al. Neuroprotection by Spice-Derived Nutraceuticals: You Are What You Eat! Mol Neurobiol., 2011; 44(2); p.142–159.

[461] Shukla Y, Singh M. Cancer preventive properties of ginger: A brief review. Food and Chemical Toxicology, 2007; Volume 45, Issue 5; p. 683–690.

[462] Hung JY, et al. 6-Shogaol, an Active Constituent of Dietary Ginger, Induces Autophagy by Inhibiting the AKT/mTOR Pathway in Human Non-Small Cell Lung Cancer A549 Cells. J. Agric. Food Chem., 2009; 57 (20); p. 9809–9816.

[463] Saraswat M, et al. Prevention of non-enzymic glycation of proteins by dietary agents: prospects for alleviating diabetic complications. British Journal of Nutrition, 2009; 101; p. 1714–1721.

[464] Burns J, et al. Plant Foods and Herbal Sources of Resveratrol. J. Agric. Food Chem., 2002; 50; p. 3337-3340.

[465] Catalgol B, Batirel S, Taga Y and Kartal Ozer N. Resveratrol: French paradox revisited. Front. Pharmacol., 2012; doi: 10.3389/fphar.2012.00141.

[466] Mythri RB, et al. "Therapeutic Potential of Polyphenols in Parkinson's Disease," in: Towards New Therapies for Parkinson's Disease, ed. by David Finkelstein, InTech, 2011, p. 115-150.

[467] Hershkovits AZ, Guarente L. Sirtuin deacetylases in neurodegenerative diseases of aging. Cell Research, 2013; 23; p.746-758.

[468] Zhou H, Luo Y, Huang S. Updates of mTOR inhibitors. Anticancer Agents Med Chem, 2010; 10(7); p. 571-581.

[469] Karuppagounder SS, et al. Dietary supplementation with resveratrol reduces plaque pathology in a transgenic model of Alzheimer's Disease. Neurochem Int. 2009; 54(2); p. 111–118.

[470] Dohadwala MM, Vita JA. Grapes and Cardiovascular Disease. J. Nutr., 2009; vol. 139, no. 9; p. 1788S-1793S.

[471] Zbarsky V, et al. Neuroprotective properties of the natural phenolic antioxidants curcumin and naringenin but not quercetin and fisetin in a 6-OHDA model of Parkinson's disease. Free Radical Research, 2005, Vol. 39, No. 10, Pages 1119-1125.

[472] Jung UJ, Leem E, Kim SR. Naringin: A Protector of the Nigrostriatal Dopaminergic Projection. Exp Neurobiol., 2014; 23(2); p.124-129.

[473] Bernardo D, et al. Ascorbate-dependent decrease of the mucosal immune inflammatory response to gliadin in coeliac disease patients. Allergol Immunopathol (Madr). 2012;40(1); p.3-8.

[474] Niture SK, Refai L. Plant pectin: A potential source for cancer suppression. Am. J. Pharmacol. Toxicol., 2013; 8; p. 9-19.

[475] David LA, et al. Host lifestyle affects human microbiota on daily timescales. Genome Biology, 2014; 15, R89; 15 pages.

[476] Sokol H, et al. *Faecalibacterium prausnitzii* is an anti-inflammatory commensal bacterium identified by gut microbiota analysis of Crohn disease patients. PNAS, 2008; vol. 105, no. 43; p. 16731-16736.

[477] Pirmohamed M. Drug-grapefruit juice interactions. British Medical Journal 2013; 346 doi: http://dx.doi.org/10.1136/bmj.f1.

[478] Pepe G, et al. Evaluation of anti-inflammatory activity and fast UHPLC–DAD–IT-TOF profiling of polyphenolic compounds extracted from green lettuce (Lactuca sativa L.; var. Maravilla de Verano). Food Chemistry, 2015; 167; p.153–161.

[479] Harsha SN, Anilakumar KR. Protection against aluminium neurotoxicity: A repertoire of lettuce antioxidants. Biomedicine & Aging Pathology, 2013; Volume 3, Issue 4; p.179-184.

[480] Rhee HJ, Kim EJ, Lee JK. Physiological polyamines: simple primordial stress molecules. J. Cell. Mol. Med., 2007; Vol 11, No 4; p. 685-703.

[481] Atiya Ali M, Poortvliet E, Strömberg R, Yngve A. Polyamines in foods: development of a food database. Food Nutr Res. 2011 Jan 14;55. doi: 10.3402/fnr.v55i0.5572.

[482] Phan CW, et al. Therapeutic potential of culinary-medicinal mushrooms for the management of neurodegenerative diseases: diversity, metabolite, and mechanism. Critical Reviews in Biotechnology, 2014; doi:10.3109/07388551.2014.887649.

[483] Casarejos MJ, et al. The accumulation of neurotoxic proteins, induced by proteasome inhibition, is reverted by trehalose, an enhancer of autophagy, in human neuroblastoma cells. Neurochem Int., 2011;58(4); p.512-520.

[484] Obata T. Phytic acid suppresses 1-methyl-4-phenylpyridinium ion-induced hydroxyl radical generation in rat striatum. Brain Research, 2003; Volume 978, Issues 1–2; p. 241–244.

[485] De Stefano C, Milea D, Porcino N, Sammartano S. Speciation of phytate ion in aqueous solution. Sequestering ability toward mercury(II) cation in NaClaq at different ionic strengths. J Agric Food Chem., 200654(4); p. 1459-1466.

[486] Willis LM, Bielinski DF, Fisher DR, Matthan NR, Joseph JA. Walnut extract inhibits LPS-induced activation of BV-2 microglia via internalization of TLR4: possible involvement of phospholipase D2. Inflammation,2010; 33(5); p.325-333.

[487] Poulose SM, Bielinski DF, Shukitt-Hale B. Walnut diet reduces accumulation of polyubiquitinated proteins and inflammation in the brain of aged rats. The Journal of Nutritional Biochemistry, 2013; Volume 24, Issue 5; p. 912–919.

[488] Rajesha J, et al. Antioxidant Potentials of Flaxseed by in Vivo Model. J Agric Food Chem., 2006; 54(11); p.3794-3799.

[489] Jeng KCG, Hou RCW. Sesamin and Sesamolin: Nature's Therapeutic Lignans. Current Enzyme Inhibition, 2005, 1; p. 11-20.

[490] Chandrasekaran VR, Hsu DZ, Liu MY. Beneficial effect of sesame oil on heavy metal toxicity. JPEN J Parenter Enteral Nutr., 2014; 38(2); p.179-185.

[491] Angeline SM, et al. Sesamol and naringenin reverse the effect of rotenone-induced PD rat model. Neuroscience, 2013, Volume 254; p. 379–394.

[492] Caramia G, Gori A, Valli E, Cerretani L. Virgin olive oil in preventive medicine: From legend to epigenetics. European Journal of Lipid Science and Technology, 2012, Volume 114, Issue 4, pages 375–388.

[493] Kim MS, et al. Olea europaea Linn (Oleaceae) Fruit Pulp Extract Exhibits Potent Antioxidant Activity and Attenuates Neuroinflammatory Responses in Lipopolysaccharide-Stimulated Microglial Cells. Tropical Journal of Pharmaceutical Research, 2013; 12 (3); p. 357-362.

[494] Massaro M, Carluccio MA, De Caterina R. Direct vascular antiatherogenic effects of oleic acid: a clue to the cardioprotective effects of the Mediterranean diet. Cardiologia, 1999; 44(6); p. 507-513.

[495] Andersson U, Tracey KJ. Neural reflexes in inflammation and immunity. J. Exp. Med., 2012; Vol. 209, No. 6; p. 1057-1068.

[496] Charles RL, et al. Protection from hypertension in mice by the Mediterranean diet is mediated by nitro fatty acid inhibition of soluble epoxide hydrolase. Proceedings of the National Academy of Sciences, 2014; doi: 10.1073/pnas.1402965111.

[497] Li W, et al. Inhibition of tau fibrillization by oleocanthal via reaction with the amino groups of tau. J Neurochem. 2009; 110(4); p.1339–1351.

[498] Katsiki M, et al. The olive constituent oleuropein exhibits proteasome stimulatory properties in vitro and confers life span extension of human embryonic fibroblasts. Rejuvenation Res., 2007;10(2); p.157-172.

[499] Kostomoiri M, et al. Oleuropein, an anti-oxidant polyphenol constituent of olive promotes α-secretase cleavage of the amyloid precursor protein (AβPP). Cell Mol Neurobiol., 2013; 33(1); p.147-154.

[500] Oh SH, et al. Dihydrocapsaicin (DHC), a saturated structural analog of capsaicin, induces autophagy in human cancer cells in a catalase-regulated manner. Autophagy, 2008;4(8); p.1009-1019.

[501] Mythri RB, Harish G, Bharath MM. Therapeutic potential of natural products in Parkinson's disease. Recent Pat Endocr Metab Immune Drug Discov. 2012;6(3); p.181-200.

[502] Bhui K, Tyagi S, Prakash B, Shukla Y. Pineapple bromelain induces autophagy, facilitating apoptotic response in mammary carcinoma cells. Biofactors, 2010;36(6); p. 474-482.

[503] Sindhu P, Darshan R, Shyam P, Lingaraju H. Neuroprotective Property of Bromelain on Focal Ischemia and Reperfusion Induced Cerebral Injury in Rats. Indo American Journal of Pharmaceutical Research, 2013; 3, 7; p. 5329-5341.

[504] Chintharlapalli S, Papineni S, Ramaiah SK, Safe S. Betulinic acid inhibits prostate cancer growth through inhibition of specificity protein transcription factors. Cancer Res. 2007;67(6); p.2816-2823.

[505] Park JA, et al. Beneficial effects of carnosic acid on dieldrin-induced dopaminergic neuronal cell death. Cellular, Molecular and Developmental Neuroscience, 2008; Volume 19, Issue 13; p.1301-1304.

[506] Tardiff DF, Lindquist S. Phenotypic screens for compounds that target the cellular pathologies underlying Parkinson's Disease. Drug Discov Today Technol., 2013 ; 10(1); e121–e128.

[507] Ben Jemia M, et al. NMR-based quantification of rosmarinic and carnosic acids, GC–MS profile and bioactivity relevant to neurodegenerative disorders of Rosmarinus officinalis L. extracts. Journal of Functional Foods, 2013; Volume 5, Issue 4; p.1873–1882.

[508] Kelsey NA, Wilkins HM, Linseman DA. Nutraceutical antioxidants as novel neuroprotective agents. Molecules. 2010;15(11); p. 7792-7814.

[509] Petersen M, Simmonds MS. Rosmarinic acid. Phytochemistry,2003; 62(2); p.121-125.

[510] Ono K, Yamada M. Antioxidant compounds have potent anti-fibrillogenic and fibril-destabilizing effects for alpha-synuclein fibrils in vitro. J Neurochem., 2006; 97(1); p.105-115.

[511] Romo-Vaquero M, et al. A Rosemary Extract Rich in Carnosic Acid Selectively Modulates Caecum Microbiota and Inhibits b-Glucosidase Activity, Altering Fiber and Short Chain Fatty Acids Fecal Excretion in Lean and Obese Female Rats. PLOS One, 2014; Volume 9, Issue 4, e94687.

[512] Wang X, et al. Genistein protects dopaminergic neurons by inhibiting microglial activation. Neuroreport, 2005; Volume 16, Issue 3; p.267-270.

[513] Zhao B. Natural Antioxidants Protect Neurons in Alzheimer's Disease and Parkinson's Disease. Neurochem Res., 2009; 34; p. 630–638.

[514] White LR, et al. Brain Aging and Midlife Tofu Consumption. Journal of the American College of Nutrition, 2000; Vol. 19, No. 2; p. 242–255.

[515] Barbeau A, et al. Effect of a magnesium-deficient diet on the striatal content of amines in the dog. Experientia, 1972; Volume 28, Issue 3; p. 289-291.

[516] Kubota T, et al. Mitochondria are intracellular magnesium stores: investigation by simultaneous fluorescent imagings in PC12 cells. Biochimica et Biophysica Acta, 2005; 1744; p. 19–28.

[517] Durlach J, et al. Are age-related neurodegenerative diseases linked with various types of magnesium depletion? Magnesium Research, 1997; 10(4); p. 339-353.

[518] Uitti RJ, et al. Regional metal concentrations in Parkinson's disease, other chronic neurological diseases, and control brains. Can J Neurol Sci. 1989;16(3); p.310-314.

[519] Hashimoto T, et al. Magnesium exerts both preventive and ameliorating effects in an in vitro rat Parkinson disease model involving 1-methyl-4-phenylpyridinium (MPP+) toxicity in dopaminergic neurons. Brain Research, 2008, Volume 1197; p. 143–151.

[520] Timiras PS, Hudson DB, Segall PE. Lifetime brain serotonin: regional effects of age and precursor availability. Neurobiol Aging, 1984l; 5(3); p.235-242.

[521] Cartford MC, Gemma C, Bickford PC. Eighteen-Month-Old Fischer 344 Rats Fed a Spinach-Enriched Diet Show Improved Delay Classical Eyeblink Conditioning and Reduced Expression of Tumor Necrosis Factor α (TNFα) and TNFβ in the Cerebellum. The Journal of Neuroscience, 2002;22(14); p.5813-5816.

[522] http://nutritiondata.self.com/foods-000112000000000000000.html Accessed November 6, 2014.

[523] Zeisel SH. Is there a new component of the Mediterranean diet that reduces inflammation? Am J Clin Nutr., 2008;87; p.277–278.

[524] Philippu A, Matthaei H, Lentzen H. Uptake of dopamine into fractions of pig caudate nucleus homogenates. Naunyn Schmiedebergs Arch Pharmacol., 1975; 287(2); p.181-190.

[525] Golts N, et al. Magnesium Inhibits Spontaneous and Iron-induced Aggregation of alpha-Synuclein. The Journal of Biological Chemistry, 2002; Vol. 277, No. 18; p. 16116–16123.

[526] Regan RF, Guo Y. Magnesium deprivation decreases cellular reduced glutathione and causes oxidative neuronal death in murine cortical cultures. Brain Res., 2001;890(1); p.177-183.

[527] Gao F, et al. Magnesium sulfate provides neuroprotection in lipopolysaccharide-activated primary microglia by inhibiting NF-κB pathway. J Surg Res., 2013;184(2); p.944-950.

[528] Yang UJ, et al. Water spinach (Ipomoea aquatic Forsk.) reduced the absorption of heavy metals in an in vitro bio-mimicking model system. Food and Chemical Toxicology, 2012; Volume 50, Issue 10; p. 3862–3866.

[529] Weinreb O, Mandel S, Amit T, Youdim MB. Neurological mechanisms of green tea polyphenols in Alzheimer's and Parkinson's diseases. Journal of Nutritional Biochemistry, 2004;15(9); p.506-516.

[530] Li FJ, Ji HF, Shen L. A Meta-Analysis of Tea Drinking and Risk of Parkinson's Disease. The Scientific World Journal, Volume 2012, Article ID 923464, p. 1-6.

[531] Liu X, et al. Green tea polyphenols alleviate early BBB damage during experimental focal cerebral ischemia through regulating tight junctions and PKCalpha signaling. BMC Complement Altern Med., 2013; 13; 187. doi:10.1186/1472-6882-13-187.

[532] Zhou H, Luo Y, Huang S. Updates of mTOR inhibitors. Anticancer Agents Med Chem, 2010; 10(7); p. 571-581.

[533] Mounsey RB, Teismann P. Chelators in the Treatment of Iron Accumulation in Parkinson's Disease. International Journal of Cell Biology, Volume 2012, Article ID 983245, p. 1-12.

[534] Kumazawa T, et al. Levels of pyrroloquinoline quinone in various foods. Biochem. J., 1995;307; p. 331-333.

[535] Sekiyama K, et al. Theaflavins stimulate autophagic degradation of α-synuclein in neuronal cells. Open Journal of Neuroscience, 2012; 2; p. 1-9.

[536] Keenan EK, et al. How much theanine in a cup of tea? Effects of tea type and method of preparation. Food Chemistry, 2011, Volume 125, Issue 2; p. 588–594.

[537] Cho HS, et al. Protective effect of the green tea component, L-theanine on environmental toxins-induced neuronal cell death. Neurotoxicology. 2008, 29(4); p. 656-62.

[538] Egashira N, et al. Neuroprotective effect of gamma-glutamylethylamide (theanine) on cerebral infarction in mice. Neurosci Lett., 2004; 363(1); p.58-61.

[539] Nathan PJ, Lu K, Gray M, Oliver C. The neuropharmacology of L-theanine(N-ethyl-L-glutamine): a possible neuroprotective and cognitive enhancing agent. J Herb Pharmacother. 2006;6(2); p.21-30.

[540] Muroi H, Kubo I. Combination effects of antibacterial compounds in green tea flavor against Streptococcus mutans. J. Agric. Food Chem., 1993; 41 (7); p. 1102–1105.

[541] Abd Allah AA, Ibrahium MI, Al-atrouny AM. Effect of Black Tea on Some Cariogenic Bacteria. World Applied Sciences Journal, 2011; 12 (4); p. 552-558.

[542] Subramaniam P, Eswara U, Maheshwar Reddy KR. Effect of different types of tea on Streptococcus mutans: an in vitro study. Indian J Dent Res. 2012;23(1); p.43-48.

[543] Anandhan A, Janakiraman U, Manivasagam T. Theaflavin ameliorates behavioral deficits, biochemical indices and monoamine transporters expression against subacute 1-methyl-4-phenyl-1,2,3,6-tetrahydropyridine (MPTP)-induced mouse model of Parkinson's disease. Neuroscience, 2012; Volume 218; p. 257–267.

[544] Peng S, Zhang G. Influence of Tea Polyphenols on the Formation of Advanced Glycation End Products (AGEs) in vitro and in vivo. Journal of Food and Nutrition Research, 2014; vol. 2, no. 8; p. 524-531.

[545] Di Matteo V, et al. Intake of tomato-enriched diet protects from 6-hydroxydopamine-induced degeneration of rat nigral dopaminergic neurons. J Neural Transm Suppl., 2009; (73); p. 333-341.

[546] D'Evoli L, Lombardi-Boccia G, Lucarini M. Influence of Heat Treatments on Carotenoid Content of Cherry Tomatoes. Foods, 2013; 2; p.352-363.

[547] Tang FY, Cho HJ, Pai MH, Chen YH. Concomitant supplementation of lycopene and eicosapentaenoic acid inhibits the proliferation of human colon cancer cells. J Nutr Biochem., 2009; 20(6); p.426-434.

[548] Kiho T, et al. Tomato Paste Fraction Inhibiting the Formation of Advanced Glycation End-products. Bioscience, Biotechnology, and Biochemistry, 2004; Volume 68, Issue 1; p. 200-205.

[549] Sarkar S, et al. Lithium induces autophagy by inhibiting inositol monophosphatase. The Journal of Cell Biology, 2005; vol. 170, no. 7; p. 1101-1111.

[550] Kim YH, Rane A, Lussier S, Andersen JK. Lithium protects against oxidative stress-mediated cell death in alpha-synuclein over-expressing in vitro and in vivo models of Parkinson's disease. J Neurosci Res. 2011; 89(10); p. 1666–1675.

[551] Madeo F, Eisenberg T, Kroemer G. Autophagy for the avoidance of neurodegeneration. Genes & Development, 2009; 23; p. 2253-2259.

[552] Cordeiro ML, Gundersen CB, Umbach JA. Lithium ions modulate the expression of VMAT2 in rat brain. Brain Res. 2002; 953(1-2); p.189-194.

[553] Muñoz-Montaño JR, Moreno FJ, Avila J, Diaz-Nido J. Lithium inhibits Alzheimer's disease-like tau protein phosphorylation in neurons. FEBS Lett., 1997;411(2-3); p.183-188.

[554] Gas-Pascual E, Berna A, Bach TJ, Schaller H. Plant Oxidosqualene Metabolism: Cycloartenol Synthase–Dependent Sterol Biosynthesis in Nicotiana benthamiana. PLOS ONE, 2014; DOI: 10.1371/journal.pone.0109156.

[555] Lim L, et al. Lanosterol induces mitochondrial uncoupling and protects dopaminergic neurons from cell death in a model for Parkinson's disease. Cell Death and Differentiation, 2012; 19; p. 416-427.

[556] Goldstein DS, et al. A vesicular sequestration to oxidative deamination shift in myocardial sympathetic nerves in Parkinson's disease. Journal of Neurochemistry, 2014; Volume 131, Issue 2; p. 219–228.

[557] Schofeld G, Quigley R, Brown R. Does sedentary behaviour contribute to chronic disease or chronic disease risk in adults? A report prepared by the Scientific Committee of Agencies for Nutrition Action, July 2009, New Zealand.

[558] Dunstan DW, et al. Breaking Up Prolonged Sitting Reduces Postprandial Glucose and Insulin Responses. Diabetes Care. 2012;35(5):p. 976-983.

[559] Schofeld G, Quigley R, Brown R. Does sedentary behaviour contribute to chronic disease or chronic disease risk in adults? A report prepared by the Scientific Committee of Agencies for Nutrition Action, July 2009, New Zealand.

[560] Tudor-Locke C, et al. A step-defined sedentary lifestyle index: <5000 steps/day. Appl. Physiol. Nutr. Metab. 2013, 38: p. 100–114.

[561] Elenkov IJ, Wilder RL, Chrousos GP, Vizi ES. The sympathetic nerve—an integrative interface between two supersystems: the brain and the immune system. Pharmacol Rev. 2000;52(4); p.595-638.

[562] Young DR, et al. Effects of Physical Activity and Sedentary Time on the Risk of Heart Failure. Circ Heart Fail. 2014;7; p.21-27.

[563] Heaslop MJA. The health risks associated with prolonged sitting: a systematic review. Master's thesis, University of Adelaide, 2011.

[564] Tremblay MS, et al. Physiological and health implications of a sedentary lifestyle. Appl. Physiol. Nutr. Metab. 2010, 35: p. 725–740.

[565] Ahlskog JE, et al. Physical Exercise as a Preventive or Disease-Modifying Treatment of Dementia and Brain Aging. Mayo Clin Proc., 2011;86(9); p.876-884.

[566] Pedersen BK. The Diseasome of Physical Inactivity—and the role of myokines in muscle-fat cross talk. J Physiol. 2009 Dec 1;587(Pt 23):5559-68.

[567] Hamer M, Chida Y. Physical activity and risk of neurodegenerative disease: a systematic review of prospective evidence. Psychological Medicine, 2009, Volume 39, Issue 01; p. 3-11.

[568] Elokda AS, Nielsen DH. Effects of exercise training on the glutathione antioxidant system. Eur J Cardiovasc Prev Rehabil. 2007 Oct;14(5): p. 630-637.

[569] Trejo JL, Carro E, Nuñez A, Torres-Aleman I. Sedentary life impairs self-reparative processes in the brain: the role of serum insulin-like growth factor-I. Rev Neurosci. 2002;13(4): p. 365-74.

[570] Wehrwein EA, Roskelley EM, Spitsbergen JM. GDNF is regulated in an activity-dependent manner in rat skeletal muscle. Muscle & Nerve, 2002, Volume 26, Issue 2; p. 206–211.

[571] Attwell D, et al. Glial and neuronal control of cerebral blood flow. Nature 2010; 486, 7321; p. 232-243.

[572] Snell PG, et al. Maximal vascular leg conductance in trained and untrained men. Journal of Applied Physiology February 1, 1987 vol. 62 no. 2; p. 606-610.

[573] Ritz K, van Buchem MA, Daemen MJ. The heart-brain connection: mechanistic insights and models. Neth Heart J. 2013 February; 21(2): p. 55–57.

[574] Ibid.

[575] De la Torre, JC. Cardiovascular Risk Factors Promote Brain Hypoperfusion Leading to Cognitive Decline and Dementia. Cardiovascular Psychiatry and Neurology, Volume 2012, Article ID 367516, 15 pages.

[576] Isaacson SH, Skettini, Neurogenic orthostatic hypotension in Parkinson's disease: evaluation, management, and emerging role of droxidopa. Vascular Health and Risk Management 2014:10 169–176

[577] Strbiana D, et al. The blood–brain barrier is continuously open for several weeks following transient focal cerebral ischemia. Neuroscience, 2008, Volume 153, Issue 1; p. 175–181.

[578] Cechetti F, et al. Chronic brain hypoperfusion causes early glial activation and neuronal death, and subsequent long-term memory impairment. Brain Research Bulletin 87 (2012); p. 109–116.

[579] Rodriguez-Perez AI, et al. Dopaminergic degeneration is enhanced by chronic brain hypoperfusion and inhibited by angiotensin receptor blockage. Age, 2013;35(5);1675-1690.

[580] Haia J, et al. Chronic cerebral hypoperfusion in rats causes proteasome dysfunction and aggregation of ubiquitinated proteins. Brain Research, 2011; Volume 1374; p. 73–81.

[581] Oikawa S, et al. Proteomic analysis of carbonylated proteins in the monkey substantia nigra after ischemia- reperfusion. Free Radical Research, 2014; Vol. 48, No. 6; p. 694-705.

[582] Kalaria RN. Vascular Basis for Brain Degeneration: Faltering Controls and Risk Factors for Dementia. Nutr Rev. 2010; 68(Suppl 2): p. S74–S87.

[583] de la Torre JC. Cerebromicrovascular Pathology in Alzheimer's Disease Compared to Normal Aging. Gerontology 1997;43; p.26–43.

[584] Wu X, Sun J, Li L. Chronic cerebrovascular hypoperfusion affects global DNA methylation and histone acetylation in rat brain. Neuroscience Bulletin, 2013, Volume 29, Issue 6; p. 685-692.

[585] Goldstein DS, et al. A vesicular sequestration to oxidative deamination shift in myocardial sympathetic nerves in Parkinson's disease. Journal of Neurochemistry, Volume131, Issue2, October 2014, p. 219-228.

[586] Rango M, et al. Increased brain temperature in Parkinson's disease. Clinical Neuroscience and Neuropathology, 15 February 2012 - Volume 23 - Issue 3 - p 129–133.

[587] Pathak A, et al. Heat-related morbidity in patients with orthostatic hypotension and primary autonomic failure. Mov Disorders 20(9), 2005; p. 1213-1219.

[588] Goldstein DS. Neurocardiology: Therapeutic Implications for Cardiovascular Disease. Cardiovascular Therapeutics 30 (2012) e89–e106.

[589] Matsumoto H, et al. Sudden death in Parkinson's disease: A retrospective autopsy study. Journal of the Neurological Sciences, Volume 343, Issues 1–2, 15 August 2014, Pages 149–152.

[590] Oka H, Toyoda C, Yogo M, Mochio S. Cardiovascular dysautonomia in de novo Parkinson's disease. European Journal of Neurology, 2011; 18 (2); p. 286-292.

[591] Knochel JP. Catastrophic medical events with exhaustive exercise: "White collar rhabdomyolysis." Kidney International, 1990, Vol. 38; p. 709-719.

[592] Cooper DM, et al. Dangerous exercise: lessons learned from dysregulated inflammatory responses to physical injury. J Applied Physiol, 2007; 103; p. 700-709.

[593] Suzuki K, et al. Systemic inflammatory response to exhaustive exercise. Cytokine kinetics. Exerc Immunol Rev. 2002;8; p.6-48.

[594] Ji LL, Fu R. Responses of glutathione system and antioxidant enzymes to exhaustive exercise and hydroperoxide. Journal of Applied Physiology; 1992, Vol. 72; p. 549-554.

[595] Stendig-Lindberg G, et al. Changes in serum magnesium concentration after strenuous exercise. J Am Coll Nutr. 1987;6(1); p.35-40.

[596] Hautaula A, et al. Changes in cardiac autonomic regulation after prolonged maximal exercise. Clinical Physiology, 2001; Volume 21, Issue 2; p. 238–245.

[597] Watson P, Shirreffs SM, Maughan RJ. Blood-brain barrier integrity may be threatened by exercise in a warm environment. American Journal of Physiology - Regulatory, Integrative and Comparative Physiology, 2005; Vol. 288; p. R1689-R1694.

[598] Pamphlett R, Kum Jew S. Uptake of inorganic mercury by human locus ceruleus and corticomotor neurons: implications for amyotrophic lateral sclerosis. Acta Neuropathologica Communications 2013, 1:13

[599] Armstrong LE, VanHeest JL. The Unknown Mechanism of the Overtraining Syndrome. Sports Med 2002; 32 (3); p. 185-209.

[600] Cobb LA, Weaver WD. Exercise: A risk for sudden death in patients with coronary heart disease. J Am Coll Cardiol. 1986;7(1); p.215-219.

[601] Baille G, et al. Ventilatory Dysfunction in Parkinson's Disease. Journal of Parkinson's Disease 6 (2016) p. 463-471.

[602] Bhutani N1, Burns DM, Blau HM. DNA demethylation dynamics. Cell. 2011; 146(6); p.866-872.

[603] Jowaed A1, Schmitt I, Kaut O, Wüllner U. Methylation regulates alpha-synuclein expression and is decreased in Parkinson's disease patients' brains. J Neurosci. 2010; 30(18); p.6355-6359.

[604] Barres R, et al. Acute Exercise Remodels Promoter Methylation in Human Skeletal Muscle. Cell Metabolism, 2012; Volume 15, Issue 3; p. 405–411.

[605] Ren H, et al. Epigenetic Changes in Response to Tai Chi Practice: A Pilot Investigation of DNA Methylation Marks. Evidence-Based Complementary and Alternative Medicine, 2012; Article ID 841810, 9 pages; doi:10.1155/2012/841810.

[606] Ames B, Shigenaga MK, Hagen TM. Oxidants, antioxidants, and the degenerative diseases of aging. Proc. Natl. Acad. Sci. USA, 1993, Vol. 90; p. 7915-7922.

[607] Gardiner J, Overall R, Marc J. The Nervous System under Oxidative Stress. Diseases, 2013, 1, p. 36-50.

[608] Ren Y, et al. Selective Vulnerability of Dopaminergic Neurons to Microtubule Depolymerization. J. Biol. Chem. 2005, 280:34105-34112.

[609] Bain LJ, et al. Healthy Brain Aging: A Meeting Report From The Sylvan M. Cohen Annual Retreat Of The University of Pennsylvania Institute On Aging. Alzheimers Dement. 2008 November; 4(6); p. 443–446.

[610] Ibid.

[611] Cotman CW, Berchtold NC, Christie LA. Exercise builds brain health: key roles of growth factor cascades and inflammation. TRENDS in Neurosciences Vol.30 No.9; p. 464-472.

[612] Pedersen BK, et al. Role of exercise-induced brain-derived neurotrophic factor production in the regulation of energy homeostasis in mammals. Exp Physiol. 2009 Dec;94(12); p. 1153-60.

[613] Wu SY, et al. Running exercise protects the substantia nigra dopaminergic neurons against inflammation-induced degeneration via the activation of BDNF signaling pathway. Brain, Behavior, and Immunity, 2011, Volume 25, Issue 1; p. 135–146.

[614] Saavedra A, Baltazar G, Duarte EP. Driving GDNF expression: The green and red traffic lights. Progress in Neurobiology 86 (2008); p. 186-215.

[615] Cotman CW, Berchtold NC, Christie LA. Exercise builds brain health: key roles of growth factor cascades and inflammation. TRENDS in Neurosciences Vol.30 No.9; p. 464-472.

[616] Carro E, Trejo JL, Busiguina S, Torres-Aleman I. Circulating Insulin-Like Growth Factor I Mediates the Protective Effects of Physical Exercise against Brain Insults of Different Etiology and Anatomy. The Journal of Neuroscience, 2001, 21(15); p. 5678–5684.

[617] Airavaara M, et al. CDNF protects the nigrostriatal dopamine system and promotes recovery after MPTP treatment in mice. Cell Transplant. 2012; 21(6); p. 1213–1223.

[618] Woie L, Kaada B, Opstad PK. Increase in plasma vasoactive intestinal polypeptide (VIP) in muscular exercise in humans. Gen Pharmacol. 1986;17(3); p.321-326.

[619] Hu WP, Li JD, Colwell CS, Zhou QY. Decreased REM Sleep and Altered Circadian Sleep Regulation in Mice Lacking
Vasoactive Intestinal Polypeptide. Sleep. 2011, 1;34(1); p.49-56.

[620] White CM, Ji S, Cai H, Maudsley S, Martin B. Therapeutic potential of vasoactive intestinal peptide and its receptors in neurological disorders. CNS Neurol Disord Drug Targets. 2010;9(5); p.661-666.

[621] Gozes I, et al. NAP: Research and Development of a Peptide Derived from Activity-Dependent Neuroprotective Protein (ADNP). CNS Drug Reviews, 2005; Vol. 11, No. 4; p. 353–368.

[622] Esteves AR, Gozes I, Cardoso SM. The rescue of microtubule-dependent traffic recovers mitochondrial function in Parkinson's disease. Biochim Biophys Acta, 2014;1842(1); p.7-21.

[623] Rao SSC, et al. Effects of acute graded exercise on human colonic motility. Am. J. Physiol., 1999; 276: Gastrointest. Liver Physiol. 39; p. G1221–G1226.

[624] Choi JJ, et al. Exercise Attenuates PCB-Induced Changes in the Mouse Gut Microbiome. Environmental Health Perspectives, 2013; Volume 121, Number 6; p. 725-730.

[625] Clarke SF, et al. Gut, 2013; doi:10.1136/gutjnl-2013-306541

[626] Petriz BA, et al. Exercise induction of gut microbiota modifications in obese, non-obese and hypertensive rats. BMC Genomics, 2014; 15:511; 13 pages.

[627] Mattioni M, Le Novere N. Integration of Biochemical and Electrical Signaling-Multiscale Model of the Medium Spiny Neuron of the Striatum. PLoS ONE 8(7): e66811. doi: 10.1371/journal.pone.0066811.

[628] Nagy A, et al. Multisensory integration in the basal ganglia. European Journal of Neuroscience, 2006, Vol. 24; p. 917–924.

[629] McCloskey DP, Adamo DS, Anderson BJ. Exercise increases metabolic capacity in the motor cortex and striatum, but not in the hippocampus. Brain Research 891 (2001); p. 168–175.

[630] Ouchi Y, et al. Effect of Simple Motor Performance on Regional Dopamine Release in the Striatum in Parkinson Disease Patients and Healthy Subjects: A Positron Emission Tomography Study. Journal of Cerebral Blood Flow & Metabolism (2002) 22; p. 746–752.

[631] Shon YM, et al. High frequency stimulation of the subthalamic nucleus evokes striatal dopamine release in a large animal model of human DBS neurosurgery. Neuroscience Letters, 2010, Volume 475, Issue 3; p. 136–140.

[632] Salvadore G, et al. An investigation of amino-acid neurotransmitters as potential predictors of clinical improvement to ketamine in depression. Int J Neuropsychopharmacol. 2012; 15(8); p. 1063–1072.

[633] Jia LL, et al. Exercise Training Attenuates Hypertension and Cardiac Hypertrophy by Modulating Neurotransmitters and Cytokines in Hypothalamic Paraventricular Nucleus. PLoS ONE; doi: 10.1371/journal.pone.0085481.

[634] Wilson RS, et al. Neural reserve, neuronal density in the locus ceruleus, and cognitive decline. Neurology, 2013; vol. 80, no. 13; p. 1202-1208.

[635] Hindle JV, Martyr A, Clare L. Cognitive reserve in Parkinson's disease: A systematic review and meta-analysis. Parkinsonism Relat Disord., 2013; S1353-8020(13)00304-0. doi: 10.1016/j.parkreldis.2013.08.010

[636] Stern Y. What is cognitive reserve? Theory and research application of the reserve concept. Journal of the International Neuropsychological Society, 2002; 8; p. 448–460.

[637] Robertson IH. A noradrenergic theory of cognitive reserve: implications for Alzheimer's disease. Neurobiology of Aging, 2013; Volume 34, Issue 1; p. 298-308.

[638] Steffener J, Stern Y. Exploring the neural basis of cognitive reserve in aging. Biochimica et Biophysica Acta (BBA) - Molecular Basis of Disease, 2012; Volume 1822, Issue 3; p. 467–473.

[639] Cappuccio FP, D'Elia L, Strazzullo P, Miller MA. Sleep duration and all-cause mortality: a systematic review and meta-analysis of prospective studies. Sleep, 2010;33(5); p.585-592.

[640] Donga E, et al. A Single Night of Partial Sleep Deprivation Induces Insulin Resistance in Multiple Metabolic Pathways in Healthy Subjects. J Clin Endocrinol Metab, 2010, 95(6); p.2963–2968.

[641] Dhawan V, Healy DG, Pal S, Chaudhuri KR. Sleep-related problems of Parkinson's Disease. Age and Ageing, 2006; 35; p. 220-228.

[642] Willison LD, et al. Circadian dysfunction may be a key component of the non-motor symptoms of Parkinson's disease: Insights from a transgenic mouse model. Experimental Neurology, 2013; Volume 243; p. 57–66.

[643] Videnovic A. Management of sleep disorders in Parkinson's disease and Multiple System Atrophy. Mov Disord. 2017 May; 32(5): 659–668

[644] Di Stefano C, et al. Cardiac organ damage in patients with Parkinson's disease and reverse dipping. Journal of Hypertension: February 2020 - Volume 38 - Issue 2 - p 289–294.

[645] Hornyak M, et al. Magnesium therapy for periodic leg movements-related insomnia and restless legs syndrome: an open pilot study. Sleep. 1998 Aug 1;21(5):501-5.

[646] Gomez-Gonzalez B, et al. REM Sleep Loss and Recovery Regulates Blood-Brain Barrier Function. Current Neurovascular Research, 2013, 10(3):p. 197-207.

[647] Bottum K, et al. Suprachiasmatic nucleus neurons display endogenous resistance to excitotoxicity. Exp Biol Med, 2010; Vol. 235, No. 2; p. 237-246.

[648] Kudo T, et al. Circadian dysfunction in response to the in vivo treatment with the mitochondrial toxin 3-nitropropionic acid. ASN NEURO (2013) Immediate Publication, doi:10.1042/AN20130042.

[649] Krishnan N, et al. Loss of circadian clock accelerates aging in neurodegeneration-prone mutants. Neurobiol Dis. 2012;45(3):p. 1129-1135.

[650] Anafi RC, et al. Sleep is not just for the brain: transcriptional responses to sleep in peripheral tissues. BMC Genomics, 2013; 14:362; 19 pages.

[651] Ma D, Li S, Molusky MM, Lin JD. Circadian autophagy rhythm: a link between clock and metabolism? Trends Endocrinol Metab. 2012; 23(7); p.319-325.

[652] Voight RM, et al. Circadian Disorganization Alters Intestinal Microbiota. PLOS ONE 2014; Volume 9, Issue 5; e97500, 17 pages.

[653] Cirelli C, Gutierrez CM, Tononi G. Extensive and divergent effects of sleep and wakefulness on brain gene expression. Neuron. 2004;41(1); p. 35-43.

[654] Archer S, et al. Mistimed sleep disrupts circadian regulation of the human transcriptome. Proceedings of the National Academy of Sciences. DOI: 10.1073/pnas.1316335111

[655] Mackiewicz M, et al. Macromolecule biosynthesis: a key function of sleep. Physiol. Genomics, 2007; 31; p. 441-457.

[656] Moller-Levet CS, et al. Effects of insufficient sleep on circadian rhythmicity and expression amplitude of the human blood transcriptome. doi: 10.1073/pnas.1217154110 PNAS, 2013; vol. 110 no. 12; p. E1132-E1141.

[657] Lin Q, et al. Promoter methylation analysis of seven clock genes in Parkinson's disease. Neuroscience Letters, 2012; Volume 507, Issue 2; p. 147–150.

[658] Kinoshita C, et al. Rhythmic oscillations of the microRNA miR-96-5p play a neuroprotective role by indirectly regulating glutathione levels. Nature Communications 5, 2014; Article number: 3823 doi:10.1038/ncomms4823

[659] Borelli E, et al. Decoding the Epigenetic Language of Neuronal Plasticity. Neuron, 2008, 60 (6); p. 961-974.

[660] Calegare B, Tufik S, D'Almeida V. DNA methylation and oxidative stress in sleep deprived rats. Sleep Science, 2012;5(3):p. 84-88.

[661] Mackiewicz M, et al. Macromolecule biosynthesis: a key function of sleep. Physiol Genomics, 2007; 31(3); p. 441-457.

[662] Musiek ES, et al. Circadian clock proteins regulate neuronal redox homeostasis and neurodegeneration. The Journal of Clinical Investigation, 2013; Volume 123, Number 12; p. 5389-5400.

[663] Knekt P, et al. Serum Vitamin D and the Risk of Parkinson Disease. JAMA Neurology, 2010, 67(7); p.808-811.

[664] Ramagopalan SV, et al. A ChIP-seq-defined genomewide map of vitamin D receptor binding: Associations with disease and evolution. Genome Research, 2010; DOI: 10.1101/gr.107920.110

[665] Patrick RP. Ames BN. Vitamin D hormone regulates serotonin synthesis. The FASEB Journal, 2014; vol. 28, no. 6; p.2398-2413.

[666] Ciu X, et al. The vitamin D receptor in dopamine neurons; its presence in human substantia nigra and its ontogenesis in rat midbrain. Neuroscience. 2013 Apr 16; 236:77-87.

[667] Holick MF. Sunlight, ultraviolet radiation, vitamin D and skin cancer: how much sunlight do we need? Adv Exp Med Biol., 2014;810; p.1-16.

[668] Yuk JM, et al. Vitamin D3 induces autophagy in human monocytes/macrophages via cathelicidin. Cell Host Microbe, 2009;6(3); p.231-243.

[669] Cantorna MT, et al. Vitamin D, immune regulation, the microbiota, and inflammatory bowel disease. Exp Biol Med, 2014; doi: 10.1177/1535370214523890.

[670] James LE, Asuni AA. Parkinson's Disease and the "Sunshine" Vitamin. J Alzheimers Dis Parkinsonism, 2013; 3: 120.

[671] Shipton EA, Shipton EE. Vitamin D and Pain: Vitamin D and Its Role in the Aetiology and Maintenance of Chronic Pain States and Associated Comorbidities. Pain Research and Treatment, Volume 2015, Article ID 904967

[672] Hausler MR, et al. Molecular Mechanisms of Vitamin D Action. Calcif Tissue Int. 2013;92(2); p.77-98.

[673] Zughaier SM, et al. The role of vitamin D in regulating the iron-hepcidin-ferroportin axis in monocytes. Journal of Clinical & Translational Endocrinology, 2014; Volume 1, Issue 1; p. e19–e25.

[674] Littlejohns TJ, et al. Vitamin D and the risk of dementia and Alzheimer disease. Neurology, 2014;83(10); p.920-928.

[675] Butler MW, et al. Vitamin D Receptor Gene as a Candidate Gene for Parkinson's disease. Annals of Human Genetics, 2011; 75; p. 201-210.

[676] Chan CS, Gertler TS, Surmeier DJ. Calcium homeostasis, selective vulnerability and Parkinson's disease. Trends Neurosci. 2009; 32(5); p.249-256.

[677] Juzeniene A, Moan J. Beneficial effects of UV radiation other than via vitamin D production. Dermato-Endocrinology, 2012; 4:2; p. 109–117.

[678] Bogdan C. Regulation of Lymphocytes by Nitric Oxide. In: Suppression and Regulation of Immune Responses, Methods in Molecular Biology, Volume 677, Humana Press, 2011, p. 375-393.

[679] Vincent SR. Nitric oxide neurons and neurotransmission. Progress in Neurobiology, 2010; Volume 90, Issue 2; p. 246–255.

[680] Palmer RMJ, Ferrige AG, Moncada S. Nitric oxide release accounts for the biological activity of endothelium-derived relaxing factor. Nature, 1987, 327, p. 524 – 526.

[681] Kuiper MA, et al. Decreased cerebrospinal fluid nitrate levels in Parkinson's disease, Alzheimer's disease and multiple system atrophy patients. Journal of the Neurological Sciences, 1994, Volume 121, Issue 1; p. 46–49.

[682] Torregrossa AC, Aranke M, Bryan NS. Nitric oxide and geriatrics: Implications in diagnostics and treatment of the elderly. Journal of Geriatric Cardiology, 2011, 8; p. 230–242.

[683] Pittaway JK, et al. Make Vitamin D While the Sun Shines, Take Supplements When It Doesn't: A Longitudinal, Observational Study of Older Adults in Tasmania, Australia. PLoS ONE, 2012; 8(3): e59063. doi:10.1371/journal.pone.0059063

[684] Tan D. Melatonin and the Brain. Current Neuropharmacology, 2010, Vol. 8, No. 3, p. 161.

[685] Srinivasan V, et al. Role of Melatonin in Neurodegenerative Diseases. Neurotoxicity Research, 2005, Vol. 7(4); p. 293-318.

[686] Reiter RJ, Tan DX, Fuentes- Broto, L. Melatonin: a multitasking molecule. In: Progress in Brain Research, Elsevier, 2010; p. 127-151.

[687] Sommansson, A. 2013. Regulation of Duodenal Mucosal Barrier Function and Motility. The Impact of Melatonin. Uppsala: Acta Universitatis Upsaliensis. ISBN 978-91-554-8790-4. 74 pp.

[688] Korkmaz A, Rosales-Corral S, Reiter RJ. Gene regulation by melatonin linked to epigenetic phenomena. Gene, 2012, Volume 503, Issue 1; p. 1–11.

[689] Clarke M, Crockett S, Sims B. Melatonin Induces Neuroprotection via System Xc Regulation in Neural Stem Cells. Journal of Stem Cell Research and Therapy. Volume 2, Issue 2.

[690] Lopez LC, et al. Melatonin, Neurogenesis, and Aging Brain. The Open Neuroendocrinology Journal, 2010, 3; p. 121-133.

[691] Ibid.

[692] Reiter RJ, Manchester LC, Tan DX. Neurotoxins: Free Radical Mechanisms and Melatonin Protection. Current Neuropharmacology, 2010, 8; p. 194-210.

[693] Borah A, Mohanakumar KP. Melatonin inhibits 6-hydroxydopamine production in the brain to protect against experimental parkinsonism in rodents. Journal of Pineal Research, 2009, Volume 47, Issue 4; p. 293-300.

[694] Douna H, Bavelaar BM, Pellikaan H, Olivier B, Pieters. Neuroprotection in Parkinson's Disease: A Systematic Review of the Preclinical Data. The Open Pharmacology Journal, 2012, 6, pages 12-26.

[695] Reiter R, et al. Melatonin combats molecular terrorism at the mitochondrial level. Interdisciplinary Toxicology, 2008, Volume 1 (2); p. 137-149.

[696] Lin L, Meng T, Liu T, Zheng Z. Increased melatonin may play dual roles in the striata of a 6-hydroxydopamine model of Parkinson's disease. Life Sciences, 2013, Volume 92, Issues 4–5; p. 311–316.

[697] Manda K, Reiter RJ. Melatonin maintains adult hippocampal neurogenesis and cognitive functions after irradiation. Progress in Neurobiology, 2010, Volume 90, Issue 1; p. 60–68.

[698] Tan DX, et al. Significance and application of melatonin in the regulation of brown adipose tissue metabolism: relation to human obesity. Obesity Reviews. doi: 10.1111/j.1467-789X.2010.00756.x

[699] Ono K, et al. Effect of melatonin on α-synuclein self-assembly and cytotoxicity. Neurobiology of Aging, 2012, Volume 33, Issue 9; p. 2172–2185.

[700] Mukda S, Vimolratana O, Govitrapong P. Melatonin attenuates the amphetamine-induced decrease in vesicular monoamine transporter-2 expression in postnatal rat striatum. Neurosci Lett. 2011;488(2); p.154-157.

[701] Lanfumey L, Mongeau R, Hamon M. Biological rhythms and melatonin in mood disorders and their treatments. Pharmacology & Therapeutics, 2013, Volume 138, Issue 2; 176–184.

[702] Illiff JJ, et al. A Paravascular Pathway Facilitates CSF Flow Through the Brain Parenchyma and the Clearance of Interstitial Solutes, Including Amyloid b. Sci Transl Med 4, 2012; 147ra111; p. 1-11.

[703] Francesca B, Rezzani R. Aquaporin and Blood Brain Barrier. Current Neuropharmacology, 2010, 8; p. 92-96.

[704] Fan Y, et al. Hypersensitivity of aquaporin 4-deficient mice to 1-methyl-4-phenyl-1,2,3,6-tetrahydropyrindine and astrocytic modulation. Neurobiology of Aging, 2008; Volume 29, Issue 8; p. 1226-1236.

[705] Nagelhus EA, Ottersen OP. Physiological Roles of Aquaporin-4 in brain. Physiol Rev 93, 2013; p. 1543–1562.

[706] Chi Y, et al. Novel role of aquaporin-4 in CD4+ CD25+ T regulatory cell development and severity of Parkinson's disease. Aging Cell, 2011; 10; p. 368–382.

[707] Persson L, et al. S-100 protein and neuron-specific enolase in cerebrospinal fluid and serum: markers of cell damage in human central nervous system. Stroke, 1987;18; p. 911-918.

[708] Benedict C et al. Acute sleep deprivation increases serum levels of neuron-specific enolase (NSE) and S100 calcium binding protein B (S-100B) in healthy young men. SLEEP, online 1 January 2014; DOI: 10.5665/sleep.3336.

[709] Reiter RJ. Potential biological consequences of excessive light exposure: melatonin suppression, DNA damage, cancer and neurodegenerative diseases. Neuro Endocrinol Letters, 2002; Supplement 2; p. 9-13.

[710] Yehuda S, Rabinovitz S, Mostofsk DI. Essential fatty acids and sleep: mini-review and hypothesis. Medical Hypotheses, 1998, Volume 50, Issue 2; p. 139-145.

[711] De la Puerta C, et al. Melatonin is a phytochemical in olive oil. Food Chemistry, 2007; 104; p.609–612.

[712] Iriti M, Varoni EM, Vitalini S. Melatonin in traditional Mediterranean diets. J. Pineal Res. 2010; 49; p. 101–105.

[713] Tan D. Melatonin and the Brain. Current Neuropharmacology, 2010; Vol. 8, No. 3; p. 161.

[714] Van Someren EJW, Riemersma-Van Der Lek RF. Live to the rhythm, slave to the rhythm. Sleep Medicine Reviews, 2007; 11; p. 465–484.

[715] Escames G, et al. Exercise and melatonin in humans: reciprocal benefits. Journal of Pineal Research, 2012; 52; p. 1-11.

[716] Aton SJ, et al. Vasoactive intestinal polypeptide mediates circadian rhythmicity and synchrony in mammalian clock neurons. Nat. Neurosci, 2005, 8 (4); p. 476-483.

[717] Gomez-Abellan P, Garaulet M. Adipose Tissue as a Peripheral Clock. In: Chronobiology and Obesity, Springer, 2013; p. 29-53.

[718] Nishiura c, et al. Dietary Patterns Only Partially Explain the Effect of Short Sleep Duration on the Incidence of Obesity. SLEEP, 2010, Vol. 33, No. 6; p. 753-757.

[719] Drager LF, et al. Obstructive Sleep Apnea : A Cardiometabolic Risk in Obesity and the Metabolic Syndrome. Journal of the American College of Cardiology, 2013; Volume 62, Issue 7; p. 569–576.

[720] Albrecht U. Timing to Perfection: The Biology of Central and Peripheral Circadian Clocks. Neuron, 2012, 74; p. 246-260.

[721] Giese M, et al. The Interplay of Stress and Sleep Impacts BDNF Level. PLOS ONE, 2013; Volume 8, Issue 10; p. 1-6.

[722] Hu et al. Effects of earplugs and eye masks on nocturnal sleep, melatonin and cortisol in a simulated intensive care unit environment. Critical Care 2010, 14:R66; p. 1-9.

[723] Friedman A, et al. Pyridostigmine brain penetration under stress enhances neuronal excitability and induces early immediate transcriptional response. Nat Med.,1996; 2(12); p.1382-1385.

[724] Esposito P, et al. Acute stress increases permeability of the blood–brain-barrier through activation of brain mast cells. Brain Research, 2001; 888 (1); p. 117–127.

[725] Abercrombie ED, Keefe KA, DiFrischia DS, Zigmond MA. Differential Effect of Stress on In Vivo Dopamine Release in Striatum, Nucleus Accumbens, and Medial Frontal Cortex. Journal of Neurochemistry, 1989; Volume 52, Number 5; p. 1655-1658.

[726] Sharma H, Sharma A. "Breakdown of the Blood-Brain Barrier in Stress Alters Cognitive Dysfunction and Induces Brain Pathology: New Perspectives for Neuroprotective Strategies" in: Brain Protection in Schizophrenia, Mood and Cognitive Disorders, Springer, 2010, p 243-303.

[727] Wright JW, Kawas LH, Harding JW. A role for the brain RAS in Alzheimer's and Parkinson's diseases. Frontiers in Endocrinology, 2013; Volume 4, Article 158; p. 1-12.

[728] George S, et al. Altered locus coeruleus–norepinephrine function following single prolonged stress. European Journal of Neuroscience, 2013; 37; p. 901–909.

[729] Kitayama I, et al. Degeneration of locus coeruleus axons in stress-induced depression model. Brain Research Bulletin, 1994; Volume 35, Issues 5–6; p. 573–580.

[730] Gesia M, et al. The role of the locus coeruleus in the development of Parkinson's disease. Neuroscience & Biobehavioral Reviews, 2000; Volume 24, Issue 6; p. 655–668.

[731] Ermak G, et al. Do RCAN1 proteins link chronic stress with neurodegeneration? The FASEB Journal, 2011; vol. 25, no. 10; p. 3306-3311.

[732] Luo J, et al. A calcineurin and NFAT-dependent pathway is involved in α-synuclein-induced degeneration of midbrain dopaminergic neurons. Hum. Mol. Genet. , 2014;doi: 10.1093/hmg/ddu377.

[733] Hosang GM, et al. Interaction between stress and the BDNF Val66Met polymorphism in depression: a systematic review and meta-analysis. BMC Medicine, 2014; 12:7; 11 pages.

[734] Munhoz CD, et al. Stress-induced neuroinflammation: mechanisms and new pharmacological targets. Brazilian Journal of Medical and Biological Research, 2008; 41; p.1037-1046.

[735] Snyder JS, et al. Adult hippocampal neurogenesis buffers stress responses and depressive behavior. Nature, 2011; 476; p. 458–461.

[736] Lucassen PJ, et al. Regulation of adult neurogenesis by stress, sleep disruption, exercise and inflammation: Implications for depression and antidepressant action. European Neuropsychopharmacology, 2010; 20; p. 1–17.

[737] Dhabhar FS, McEwen BS. Acute Stress Enhances while Chronic Stress Suppresses Cell-Mediated Immunity *in Vivo*: A Potential Role for Leukocyte Trafficking. Brain, Behavior, and Immunity, 1997; Volume 11, Issue 4; p. 286–306.

[738] Konturek PC, Brzozowski T, Konturek SJ. Stress and the gut: pathophysiology, clinical consequences, diagnostic approach and treatment options. J Physiol Pharmacol., 2011;62(6); p.591-599.

[739] Bhasin MK, et al. Relaxation response induces temporal transcriptome changes in energy metabolism, insulin secretion and inflammatory pathways. PLoS One. 2013;8(5): e62817.

[740] Lazar SW, et al. Meditation experience is associated with increased cortical thickness. Neuroreport, 2005; 16(17); p.1893–1897.

[741] Andersson U, Tracey KJ. Neural reflexes in inflammation and immunity. J. Exp. Med., 2012; Vol. 209, No. 6; p. 1057-1068.

[742] Smart K, et al. A potential case of remission of Parkinson's disease. J Complement Integr Med 2016; 13(3): 311–315.

[743] Melville GW, et al. Fifteen Minutes of Chair-Based Yoga Postures or Guided Meditation Performed in the Office Can Elicit a Relaxation Response. Evidence-Based Complementary and Alternative Medicine, 2012; Article ID 501986, 9 pages.

[744] Genter MB, Kendig EL, Knutson MD. Uptake of Materials from the Nasal Cavity into the Blood and Brain. International Symposium on Olfaction and Taste. Ann. N.Y. Acad. Sci., 2009; 1170; p. 623–628.

[745] Calderon-Garciduenas L, et al. Long-term Air Pollution Exposure Is Associated with Neuroinflammation, and Altered Innate Immune Response, Disruption of the Blood-Brain Barrier, Ultrafine Particulate Deposition, and Accumulation of Amyloid Beta-42 and Alpha-Synuclein in Children and Young Adults. Toxicologic Pathology, 2008; 36; p. 289-310.

[746] Calderón-Garcidueña L, et al. Air Pollution and Children: Neural and Tight Junction Antibodies and Combustion Metals, the Role of Barrier Breakdown and Brain Immunity in Neurodegeneration. J Alzheimers Dis., 2014 Aug 21. [Epub ahead of print]

[747] Calderón-Garcidueña L, et al. The impact of environmental metals in young urbanites' brains. Exp Toxicol Pathol. 2013;65(5); p.503-511.

[748] Bos I, et al. Subclinical effects of aerobic training in urban environment. Medicine and Science in Sports and Exercise, 2013; 45 (3); p. 439-447.

[749] Levesque S, Surace M, McDonald J, Block M. Air pollution & the brain: Subchronic diesel exhaust exposure causes neuroinflammation and elevates early markers of neurodegenerative disease. Journal of Neuroinflammation. 2011; 8; p. 105.

[750] Thomson EM, et al. Mapping Acute Systemic Effects of Inhaled Particulate Matter and Ozone: Multiorgan Gene Expression and Glucocorticoid Activity. Toxicological Sciences, 2013; 135(1); p. 169–181.

[751] Mutlu EA. et al. Particulate matter air pollution causes oxidant mediated increase in gut permeability in mice. Particle and Fibre Toxicology ,2011; 8:19; 13 pages.

[752] Peters A, et al. Translocation and potential neurological effects of fine and ultrafine particles a critical update. Particle and Fibre Toxicology, 2006; 3; p.13.

[753] Langston JW, Ballard P, Tetrud JW, Irwin I. Chronic Parkinsonism in humans due to a product of meperidine-analog synthesis. Science, 1983; Vol. 219, No. 4587; p. 979-980.

[754] Sherer T, et al. Mechanism of toxicity of pesticides acting at complex I: relevance to environmental etiologies of Parkinson's disease. Journal of Neurochemistry, 2007; Volume 100, Issue 6; p.1469–1479.

[755] Manning-Bog AB, et al. The Herbicide Paraquat Causes Up-regulation and Aggregation of alpha-Synuclein in Mice. The Journal of Biological Chemistry, 2002; 277; p. 1641-1644.

[756] Kanthasamy A, et al. Emerging Neurotoxic Mechanisms in Environmental Factors Induced Neurodegeneration. Neurotoxicology, 2012; 33(4); p.833–837.

[757] Mostafalou S, Abdollahi M. Pesticides and human chronic diseases: Evidences, mechanisms, and perspectives. Toxicology and Applied Pharmacology, 2013; 268; p. 157–177.

[758] Golamundi S, et al. Concordant Signaling Pathways Produced by Pesticide Exposure in Mice Correspond to Pathways Identified in Human Parkinson's Disease. PLoS ONE, 2012; Volume 7, Issue 5; p. 1-13.

[759] Tanner CM, et al. Rotenone, paraquat and Parkinson's disease. Environ Health Perspect., 2011; 119(6); 866–872.

[760] http://www.nap.edu/catalog.php?record_id=12662 Accessed August 25, 2013.

[761] Gatto NM, Cockburn M, Bronstein J, Manthripragada AD, and Ritz B. Well-Water Consumption and Parkinson's Disease in Rural California. Environmental Health Perspectives, 2009; Volume 117, Number 12; p. 1912-1919.

[762] Betarbet R, et al. Intersecting pathways to neurodegeneration in Parkinson's disease: Effects of the pesticide rotenone on DJ-1, α-synuclein, and the ubiquitin–proteasome system. Neurobiology of Disease, 2006; Volume 22, Issue 2; p. 404–420.

[763] Fernandez-Salvador, L. Use and Status of Rotenone in Organic Gardening. http://www.motherearthnews.com/organic-gardening/rotenone-organic-zb0z1405zsto.aspx Accessed March 18, 2015.

[764] Fitzmaurice AG, et al. Aldehyde dehydrogenase inhibition as a pathogenic mechanism in Parkinson disease. Proc Natl Acad Sci U S A. 2013; 110(2):p. 636–641.

[765] Dick FD, et al. Environmental risk factors for Parkinson's disease and parkinsonism: the Geoparkinson study. Occup Environ Med 2007;64; p.666–672.

[766] Butterfield PG, et al. Environmental antecedents of young-onset Parkinson's disease. Neurology, 1993. Volume 43, No. 6, p. 1150-1158.

[767] Gatto NM, Cockburn M, Bronstein J, Manthripragada AD, and Ritz B. Well-Water Consumption and Parkinson's Disease in Rural California. Environmental Health Perspectives, 2009; Volume 117, Number 12; p. 1912-1919.

[768] Lipton SA, et al. Isogenic Human iPSC Parkinson's Model Shows Nitrosative Stress-Induced Dysfunction in MEF2-PGC1α Transcription. Cell, 27 November 2013; 10.1016/j.cell.2013.11.009.

[769] Du G, et al. Microstructural changes in the substantia nigra of asymptomatic agricultural workers. Neurotoxicology and Teratology, 2014; Volume 41; p. 60–64.

[770] Kozlowski H, et al. Copper, iron, and zinc ions homeostasis and their role in neurodegenerative disorders (metal uptake, transport, distribution and regulation). Coordination Chemistry Reviews, 2009; Volume 253, Issues 21–22; p. 2665–2685.

[771] Olivieri S, et al. Ceruloplasmin Oxidation, a Feature of Parkinson's Disease CSF, Inhibits Ferroxidase Activity and Promotes Cellular Iron Retention. The Journal of Neuroscience, 2011; 31(50); p.18568 –18577.

[772] Montes S, et al. Copper and Copper Proteins in Parkinson's Disease. Oxidative Medicine and Cellular Longevity, 2014; Article ID 147251, 15 pages.

[773] Betts KS. A Study in Balance. Environmental Health Perspectives, 2011; Volume 119, Number 8; p. A340-A345.

[774] Yamin G, Glaser CB, Uversky VN, Fink AL. Certain Metals Trigger Fibrillation of Methionine-oxidized α-Synuclein. The Journal of Biological Chemistry, 2003; 78; p. 27630-27635.

[775] Uversky VN, Li J, Bower K, Fink AF. Synergistic Effects of Pesticides and Metals on the Fibrillation of a-Synuclein: Implications for Parkinson's Disease. NeuroToxicology, 2002; 23; p. 527–536.

[776] Sadiq S, Ghazala Z, Chowdhury A, Busselberg D. Metal Toxicity at the Synapse: Presynaptic, Postsynaptic, and Long-Term Effects. Journal of Toxicology; Article ID 132671, 42 pages; doi:10.1155/2012/132671.

[777] Desole MS, et al. Dopaminergic system activity and cellular defense mechanisms in the striatum and striatal synaptosomes of the rat subchronically exposed to manganese. Arch Toxicol. 1994;68(9); p. 566-70.

[778] Silva AC, Lee JH, Aoki I, Koretsky AP. Manganese-enhanced magnetic resonance imaging (MEMRI): methodological and practical considerations. NMR Biomed., 2004;17(8); p.532-543.

[779] Park RM. Neurobehavioral deficits and parkinsonism in occupations with manganese exposure: a review of methodological issues in the epidemiological literature. Saf Health Work. 2013;4(3); p.123-135.

[780] Lucchini RG, et al. High prevalence of parkinsonian disorders associated to manganese exposure in the vicinities of ferroalloy industries. American Journal of Industrial Medicine; 2007; Volume 50, Issue 11; p. 788–800.

[781] Finkelstein MM, Jerrett M. A study of the relationships between Parkinson's disease and markers of traffic-derived and environmental manganese air pollution in two Canadian cities. Environ Res., 2007;104(3):p. 420-432.

[782] Willis AW, et al. Metal Emissions and Urban Incident Parkinson Disease: A Community Health Study of Medicare Beneficiaries by Using Geographic

Information Systems. American Journal of Epidemiology, 2010, Vol. 172, No. 12, p. 1357-1363.

[783] Roels HA, et al. Manganese exposure and cognitive deficits: A growing concern for manganese neurotoxicity. Neurotoxicology. 2012; 33(4): doi: 10.1016/j.neuro.2012.03.009.

[784] http://www.atsdr.cdc.gov/toxprofiles/tp151-c6.pdf Accessed August 28, 2013.

[785] Weisskopf MG, et al. Association of Cumulative Lead Exposure with Parkinson's Disease. Environmental Health Perspectives, 2010; Volume 12, number 11, p. 1609-1613.

[786] http://www.nyc.gov/html/doh/downloads/pdf/lead/lead-fact-sheet.pdf Accessed August 28, 2013.

[787] Liu S, Hammond SK, Rojas-Cheatham A. Concentrations and Potential Health Risks of Metals in Lip Products. Environmental Health Perspectives, 2013; volume 121, number 6; p. 705-710.

[788] http://www.fda.gov/cosmetics/productandingredientsafety/productinformation/ucm137224.htm#expanalyses Accessed August 30, 2013.

[789] Ngim C, Devathasan G. Epidemiologic Study on the Association between Body Burden Mercury Level and Idiopathic Parkinson's Disease. Neuroepidemiology, 1989;8; p.128–141.

[790] Haley BE. The relationship of the toxic effects of mercury to exacerbation of the medical condition classified as Alzheimer's disease. Medical Veritas, 2007; 4; p. 1484–1498.

[791] Bartova J, et al. Dental amalgam as one of the risk factors in autoimmune diseases. Neuroendocrinology Letters, 2003; Nos. 1,2, Feb-Apr, Volume 24; p. 65-67.

[792] Azevado BF, et al. Toxic Effects of Mercury on the Cardiovascular and Central Nervous Systems. Journal of Biomedicine and Biotechnology, Volume 2012, Article ID 949048, 11 pages.

[793] Pamphlett R, Kum Jew S. Uptake of inorganic mercury by human locus ceruleus and corticomotor neurons: implications for amyotrophic lateral sclerosis. Acta Neuropathologica Communications 2013, 1:13

[794] Syversena T, Kaur P. The toxicology of mercury and its compounds. Journal of Trace Elements in Medicine and Biology, 2012; 26; p. 215–226.

[795] Xu F, et al. Mercury-induced toxicity of rat cortical neurons is mediated through N-methyl-D-Aspartate receptors. Molecular Brain 2012, 5:30.

[796] Echeverria D, et al. Chronic low-level mercury exposure, BDNF polymorphism, and associations with cognitive and motor function. Neurotoxicol Teratol. 2005;27(6); p.781-796.

[797] Guzzi G, et al. Dental Amalgam and Mercury Levels in Autopsy Tissues. Am J Forensic Med Pathol 2006; 27; p. 42–45.

[798] Rooney, J.P.K., The retention time of inorganic mercury in the brain—A systematic review of the evidence, Toxicol. Appl. Pharmacol., 2014; 274(3); p.425-435.

[799] Bondy SC. The neurotoxicity of environmental aluminum is still an issue. Neurotoxicology. 2010; 31(5); p. 575–581.

[800] Yasui M, Kihira T, Ota K. Calcium, magnesium and aluminum concentrations in Parkinson's disease. Neurotoxicology. 1992;13(3); p.593-600.

[801] Lemire J, Appanna VD. Aluminum toxicity and astrocyte dysfunction: A metabolic link to neurological disorders. Journal of Inorganic Biochemistry, 2011; 105; p. 1513–1517.

[802] Nam SM, et al. Additive or Synergistic Effects of Aluminum on the Reduction of Neural Stem Cells, Cell Proliferation, and Neuroblast Differentiation in the Dentate Gyrus of High-Fat Diet-Fed Mice. Biological Trace Element Research, 2014; Volume 157, Issue 1; p. 51-59.

[803] Gash, DM, et al. Trichloroethylene: Parkinsonism and complex 1 mitochondrial neurotoxicity. Annals of Neurology, 2008, Volume 63, Issue 2; p. 184–192.

[804] Goldman S, et al. Solvent Exposures and Parkinson's Disease Risk in Twins. Annals of Neurology, 2012; Volume 71, Issue 6; p. 776–784.

[805] http://www.atsdr.cdc.gov/toxprofiles/tp19-c5.pdf Accessed August 24, 2013.

[806] Seelbach M, et al. Polychlorinated Biphenyls Disrupt Blood–Brain Barrier Integrity and Promote Brain Metastasis Formation. Environ Health Perspect. 2010; 118(4); p. 479–484.

[807] Choi JJ et al. Lipopolysaccharide Potentiates Polychlorinated Biphenyl induced Disruption of the Blood–Brain Barrier via TLR4/IRF-3 Signaling. Toxicology, 2012; 302(2-3); p. 212–220.

[808] Hatcher-Martin JM, et al. Association between polychlorinated biphenyls and Parkinson's disease neuropathology. Neurotoxicology, 2012; 33 (5); p.1298-1304.

[809] Bradner JM, et al. Exposure to the Polybrominated Diphenyl Ether Mixture DE-71 Damages the Nigrostriatal Dopamine System: Role of Dopamine Handling in Neurotoxicity. Exp Neurol. 2013; 241; p. 138–147.

[810] Elobeid MA, et al. Endocrine Disruptors and Obesity: An Examination of Selected Persistent Organic Pollutants in the NHANES 1999–2002 Data. Int. J. Environ. Res. Public Health 2010, 7; p. 2988-3005.

[811] Alter SP, Lenzi GM, Bernstein AI, Miller GW. Vesicular integrity in Parkinson's disease. Curr Neurol Neurosci Rep. 2013;13(7):362. doi: 10.1007/s11910-013-0362-3.

[812] Ritz B, et al. Pooled analysis of tobacco use and risk of Parkinson disease. Arch Neurol. 2007;64(7); p.990-997.

[813] Miksys S, Tyndale RF. Nicotine induces brain CYP enzymes: relevance to Parkinson's disease. J Neural Transm Suppl. 2006;(70); p.177-180.

[814] Quik M, Perez XA, Bordia T. Nicotine as a potential neuroprotective agent for Parkinson's disease. Mov Disord. 2012; 27(8); p. 947–957.

[815] Hong DP, Fink AL, Uversky VN. Smoking and Parkinson's disease: does nicotine affect alpha-synuclein fibrillation? Biochim Biophys Acta. 2009;1794(2); p. 282-290.

[816] Rodgman A. Problems with the Tobacco Products Scientific Advisory Committee (TPSAC) List of Harmful or Potentially Harmful Tobacco and/or Tobacco Smoke Components. Beiträge zur Tabakforschung International/ Contributions to Tobacco Research, 2011; Volume 24, No. 6; p. 258-276.

[817] Sears ME, Kerr KJ, Bray RI. Aresnic, Cadmium, Lead, and Mercury in Sweat: A Systematic Review. Journal of Environmental and Public Health.Volume 2012, Article ID 18745, 10 pages.

[818] Papastefanou C. Radioactivity of Tobacco Leaves and Radiation Dose Induced from Smoking. Int. J. Environ. Res. Public Health, 2009; 6; p. 558-567.

[819] Pfau W, Skog K. Exposure to beta-carbolines norharman and harman. J Chromatogr B Analyt Technol Biomed Life Sci. 2004;802(1); p.115-126.

[820] Das A, et al. Smokeless Tobacco Extract (STE)-Induced Toxicity in Mammalian Cells is Mediated by the Disruption of Cellular Microtubule Network: A Key Mechanism of Cytotoxicity. PLOS One, 2013; Volume 8, Issue 7; e68224

[821] Gramage E, Herradón G. Connecting Parkinson's disease and drug addiction: common players reveal unexpected disease connections and novel therapeutic approaches. Curr Pharm Des., 2011;17(5); p.449-461.

[822] Tavassoly O, Lee JS. Methamphetamine binds to α-synuclein and causes a conformational change which can be detected by nanopore analysis. FEBS Lett., 2012;586(19); p.3222-3228.

[823] White SM, Lambe CJ. The pathophysiology of cocaine abuse. J Clin Forensic Med., 2003;10(1); p.27-39.

[824] Sulzer D, et al. Amphetamine Redistributes Dopamine from Synaptic Vesicles to the Cytosol and Promotes Reverse Transport. The Journal of Neuroscience, May 1995, 15(5): 4102-4108.

[825] Curtin K, et al. Methamphetamine/amphetamine abuse and risk of Parkinson's disease in Utah: A population-based assessment. Drug and Alcohol Dependence, 2015; Volume 146; p. 30–38.

[826] Bloomfield MAP, et al. The link between dopamine function and apathy in cannabis users: an [18F]-DOPA PET imaging study. Psychopharmacology, 2014; Volume 231, Issue 11; p. 2251-2259.

[827] Bolaños CA, Nestler EJ. Neurotrophic mechanisms in drug addiction. Neuromolecular Med. 2004;5(1); p.69-83.

[828] Sulzer D. How Addictive Drugs Disrupt Presynaptic Dopamine Neurotransmission. Neuron, 2011; 69(4); p. 628–649.

[829] Selikhova M, et al. Parkinsonism and dystonia caused by the illicit use of ephedrone—a longitudinal study. Mov Disord., 2008;23(15); p.2224-2231.

[830] Brenner DJ, Hall EJ. Computed tomography—an increasing source of radiation exposure. N Engl J Med., 2007;357(22); p.2277-2284.

[831] Ibid.

[832] Kempf SJ, Azimzadeh O, Atkinson MJ, Tapio S. Long-term effects of ionising radiation on the brain: cause for concern? Radiat Environ Biophys., 2013;52(1); p. 5-16.

[833] Ibid.

[834] Momcilovic B, et al. Environmental radon daughters reveal pathognomonic changes in the brain proteins and lipids in patients with Alzheimer's disease and Parkinson's disease, and cigarette smokers. Arh Hig Rada Toksikol., 1999; 50 (4); p. 347-369.

[835] Manicelli F, et al. Non-thermal effects of electromagnetic fields at mobile phone frequency on the refolding of an intracellular protein: Myoglobin. Journal of Cellular Biochemistry, 2004; Volume 93, Issue 1; p. 188-196.

[836] Celik MS, et al. Extremely low-frequency magnetic field induces manganese accumulation in brain, kidney and liver of rats. Toxicology and Industrial Health, 2013; doi: 10.1177/07482337134802014

[837] Boscolo P, Iovene R, Paiardini G. Electromagnetic fields and autoimmune diseases. Prevention and Research, 2014; 3(2); p. 79–83.

[838] Halgamuge MN. Pineal melatonin level disruption in humans due to electromagnetic fields and ICNIRP limits; Radiation Protection Dosimetry, 2013; Vol. 154, No. 4; p. 405-416.

[839] Reale M, et al. Neuronal Cellular Responses to Extremely Low Frequency Electromagnetic Field Exposure: Implications Regarding Oxidative Stress and Neurodegeneration. PLoS ONE, 2014;9(8): e104973. doi: 10.1371/journal.pone.0104973.

[840] Cao H, et al. Circadian Rhythmicity of Antioxidant Markers in Rats Exposed to 1.8 GHz Radiofrequency Fields. Int. J. Environ. Res. Public Health, 2015; 12; p. 2071-2087.

[841] Nitby H, et al. Increased blood-brain barrier permeability in mammalian brain 7 days after exposure to the radiation from a GSM-900 mobile phone. Pathophysiology, 2009; 16; p. 103-112.

[842] Meral I, et al. Effects of 900-MHz electromagnetic field emitted from cellular phone on brain oxidative stress and some vitamin levels of guinea pigs. Brain Res., 2007;1169; p.120-124

[843] Aboul Ezz HS, et al. The effect of pulsed electromagnetic radiation from mobile phone on the levels of monoamine neurotransmitters in four different areas of rat brain. Eur Rev Med Pharmacol Sci., 2013;17(13); p.1782-1788.

[844] Ali KJ, Hasan GT, Husain MK. Measurement of the SAR Levels Near the Human Head for Different Types of Mobile Phone device. Aust. J. Basic & Appl. Sci., 2014; 8(9); p. 130-134.

[845] Porta M, Zumeta E. Implementing the Stockholm Treaty on Persistent Organic Pollutants. Occup Environ Med 2002;59; p. 651–653.

[846] Furlong M, et al. Protective glove use and hygiene habits modify the associations of specific pesticides with Parkinson's disease. Environment International, 2015; Volume 75; p. 144–150.

[847] Fan S, et al. DIM (3,3'-diindolylmethane) confers protection against ionizing radiation by a unique mechanism. Proc Natl Acad Sci U S A., 2013;110(46); p.18650-18655.

[848] Reiter RJ, et al. Melatonin protection from chronic, low-level ionizing radiation. Mutation Research/Reviews in Mutation Research, 2012; Volume 751, Issue 1; p. 7–14.

[849] http://www.cdc.gov/nchs/fastats/obesity-overweight.htm Accessed July 10. 2014.

[850] http://www.euro.who.int/en/health-topics/noncommunicable-diseases/obesity/data-and-statistics Accessed July 10, 2014.

[851] Andersson U, Tracey KJ. Neural reflexes in inflammation and immunity. J. Exp. Med., 2012; Vol. 209, No. 6; p. 1057-1068.

[852] Zhang P, Tian B. Metabolic Syndrome: An Important Risk Factor for Parkinson's Disease. Oxidative Medicine and Cellular Longevity,2014, Article ID 729194, 7 pages.

[853] Petersen AMW, Pedersen BK. The anti-inflammatory effect of exercise. J Appl Physiol, 2005; 98; p. 1154-1162.

[854] Andersen HH, Johnsen KB, Moos T. Iron deposits in the chronically inflamed central nervous system and contributes to neurodegeneration. Cell. Mol. Life. Sci., 2014, 71; p. 1607-1622.

[855] Olmos G, Llado J. Tumor Necrosis Factor Alpha: A Link between Neuroinflammation and Excitotoxicity. Mediators of Inflammation, 2014; Article ID 861231, 12 pages.

[856] Chertoff M, et al. Neuroprotective and neurodegenerative effects of the chronic expression of tumor necrosis factor α in the nigrostriatal dopaminergic circuit of adult mice. Experimental Neurology, 2011, 227; p. 237–251.

[857] Kim MJ, et al. Fate and Complex Pathogenic Effects of Dioxins and Polychlorinated Biphenyls in Obese Subjects before and after Drastic Weight Loss. Environmental Health Perspectives, 2011; Volume 119, Number 3; p. 377-383.

[858] Elobeid MA; et al. Endocrine Disruptors and Obesity: An Examination of Selected Persistent Organic Pollutants in the NHANES 1999–2002 Data. Int. J. Environ. Res. Public Health, 2010; 7; p. 2988-3005.

[859] Kessler RM, et al. Changes in Dopamine Release and Dopamine D2/3 Receptor Levels with the Development of Mild Obesity. Synapse, 2014; 68; p. 317-320.

[860] Ouyang S, et al. Diet-induced obesity suppresses expression of many proteins at the blood–brain barrier. Journal of Cerebral Blood Flow & Metabolism, 2014; 34; p. 43–51.

[861] Velloso LA, Schwartz MW. Altered hypothalamic function in diet-induced obesity. Int J Obes (Lond), 2011; 35(12); p.1455–1465.

[862] Tanner JM, et al. Prevalence of Comorbid Obstructive Sleep Apnea and Metabolic Syndrome: Syndrome Z and Maxillofacial Surgery Implications. J Oral Maxillofac Surg., 2012; 70; p. 179-187.

[863] Daulatzai MA. Quintessential Risk Factors: Their Role in Promoting Cognitive Dysfunction and Alzheimer's Disease. Neurochemical Research, 2012; Volume 37, Issue 12; p. 2627-2658.

[864] Verstynen TD, et al. Increased Body Mass Index Is Associated With a Global and Distributed Decrease in White Matter Microstructural Integrity. Psychosom Med. 2012; 74(7); p. 682–690.

[865] Barker RA, Cahn AP. Parkinson's disease: An Autoimmune Process. International Journal of Neuroscience, 1988; Vol. 43, No. 1-2; p. 1-7.

[866] Cebrian C, et al. MHC-I expression renders catecholaminergic neurons susceptible to T-cell-mediated degeneration. Nature Communications, 2014; 5, Article number: 3633 doi:10.1038/ncomms4633

[867] Nicolson GL. Chronic Bacterial and Viral Infections in Neurodegenerative and Neurobehavioral Diseases. Labmedicine, 2008; Volume 39, Number 5; p. 291-299.

[868] Rohn TT, Catlin LW. Immunolocalization of Influenza A Virus and Markers of Inflammation in the Human Parkinson's Disease Brain. PLoS ONE, 2011; Volume 6, Issue 5; e20495; 10 pages.

[869] Jang H, et al. Highly pathogenic H5N1 influenza virus can enter the central nervous system and induce neuroinflammation and neurodegeneration. PNAS, 2009; vol. 106, no. 33; p. 14063-14068.

[870] Bobyn J, et al. Viral-toxin interactions and Parkinson's disease: poly(I:C) priming enhanced the neurodegenerative effects of paraquat. Journal of Neuroinflammation, 2012; 9:86; 10 pages.

[871] Talan J. COVID-19: Neurologists in Italy to Colleagues in US: Look for Poorly-Defined Neurologic Conditions in Patients with the Coronavirus. https://journals.lww.com/neurotodayonline/blog/breaking-news/pages/post.aspx?PostID=920 Accessed April 11, 2020.

[872] Reichling DB, Levine JD. Pain and death: Neurodegenerative disease mechanisms in the nociceptor. Ann Neurol. 2011; 69; p. 13–21.

[873] Rodriguez-Raecke R, et al. Brain Gray Matter Decrease in Chronic Pain Is the Consequence and Not the Cause of Pain. The Journal of Neuroscience, 2009;29(44); p. 13746-13750.

[874] Geha PY, et al. The Brain in Chronic CRPS Pain: Abnormal Gray-White Matter Interactions in Emotional and Autonomic Regions. Neuron, 2008; 60; p. 570–581.

[875] Brooks TA, et al. Chronic inflammatory pain leads to increased blood-brain barrier permeability and tight junction protein alterations. Am J Physiol Heart Circ Physiol, 2005; 289; p. H738–H743.

[876] Edwards RR, et al. Sleep continuity and architecture: associations with pain-inhibitory processes in patients with temporomandibular joint disorder. Eur J Pain. 2009;13(10); p.1043-1047.

[877] Shaw IR, et al. Acute Intravenous Administration of Morphine Perturbs Sleep Architecture in Healthy Pain-Free Young Adults: a Preliminary Study. SLEEP, 2005; Vol. 28, No. 6; p. 677-682.

[878] Shipton EA, Shipton EE. Vitamin D and Pain: Vitamin D and Its Role in the Aetiology and Maintenance of Chronic Pain States and Associated Comorbidities. Pain Research and Treatment, Volume 2015, Article ID 904967, 12 pages.

[879] Cicciù M, Risitano G, Lo Giudice G, Bramanti E. Periodontal Health and Caries Prevalence Evaluation in
Patients Affected by Parkinson's Disease. Parkinsons Dis., 2012;2012:541908. doi: 10.1155/2012/541908.

[880] David LA, et al. Host lifestyle affects human microbiota on daily timescales. Genome Biology, 2014; 15; R89; 15 pages.

[881] Ibid.

[882] Nakano K, Nomura R, Ooshima T. Streptococcus mutans and cardiovascular diseases. Japanese Dental Science Review, 2008; 44; p. 29-37.

[883] Hattori M, et al. Effect of tea polyphenols on glucan synthesis by glucosyltransferase from Streptococcus mutans. Chemical & Pharmaceutical Bulletin, 1990; 38(3); p.717-720.

[884] Shin HW, Chung SJ. Drug-Induced Parkinsonism. J Clin Neurol., 2012;8(1);p.15-21.

[885] Jiménez-Jiménez FJ, et al. Drug-induced parkinsonism in a movement disorders unit: A four-year survey. Parkinsonism Relat Disord., 1996;2(3); p.145-149.

[886] Bondon-Guitton E, et al. Drug-induced parkinsonism: A review of 17 years' experience in a regional pharmacovigilance center in France. Movement Disorders, 2011; Volume 26, Issue 12; p. 2226–2231.

[887] Csoti I, et al. Parkinson's disease between internal medicine and neurology. J Neural Transm (2016) 123:3-17.

[888] Hogan DB, Kwan M. Patient sheet: Tips for avoiding problems with polypharmacy. CMAJ, 2006; vol. 175, no. 8; p. 876.

[889] Gleeson M, et al. The anti-inflammatory effects of exercise: mechanisms and implications for the prevention and treatment of disease. Nature Reviews Immunology, 2011; 11; p. 607-615.

[890] http://www.cdc.gov/traumaticbraininjury/pdf/BlueBook_factsheet-a.pdf Accessed July 31, 2013.

[891] http://www.cdc.gov/concussion/signs_symptoms.html Accessed July 31, 2013.

[892] Greve MW, Zink BJ. Pathophysiology of Traumatic Brain Injury. Mount Sinai Journal of Medicine, 2009; 76; p. 97-104.

[893] Chobodski A, Zink B, Szmydynger-Chodobska J. Blood-brain barrier pathophysiology in traumatic brain injury. Transl Stroke Res. 2011; 2(4) p. 492–516.

[894] Schoknecht K, Shalev H. Blood-brain barrier dysfunction in brain diseases: Clinical experience. Epilepsia, 2012, 53 (suppl. 6); p. 7-13.

[895] Werner C, Engelhard K. Pathophysiology of traumatic brain injury. British Journal of Anesthesia, 2007; 99 (1); p. 4-9.

[896] McIntosh TK, Yu T, Gennarelli TA. Alterations in Regional Brain Catecholamine Concentrations After Experimental Brain Injury in the Rat. Journal of Neurochemistry,1994; Vol. 63, Issue 4; p. 1426-1433.

[897] Hutson CB, et al. Traumatic Brain Injury in Adult Rats Causes Progressive Nigrostriatal Dopaminergic Cell Loss and Enhanced Vulnerability to the Pesticide Paraquat. Journal of Neurotrauma 2011; 28:9; p. 1783-1801.

[898] Prins M, Greco T, Alexander D, Giza CC. The pathophysiology of traumatic brain injury at a glance. Disease Models & Mechanisms, 2013; 6; p. 1-9.

[899] Ibid.

[900] Acosta SA, et al. Alpha-synuclein as a Pathological Link between Chronic Traumatic Brain Injury and Parkinson's disease. Journal of cellular Physiology, 2014; DOI: 10.1002/jcp.24830

[901] Bansal V, et al. Traumatic Brain Injury and Intestinal Dysfunction: Uncovering the Neuro-Enteric Axis. Journal of Neurotrauma, 2009; 26; p.1353–1359

[902] Hang CH, et al. Alterations of intestinal mucosa structure and barrier function following traumatic brain injury in rats. World J Gastroenterol. 2003;9(12); p.2776-81.

[903] Andersson U, Tracey KJ. Neural reflexes in inflammation and immunity. J. Exp. Med., 2012; Vol. 209, No. 6; p. 1057-1068.

[904] http://www.cdc.gov/HomeandRecreationalSafety/Falls/index.html Accessed November 1, 2013.

905 Allen NE, Schwarzel AK, Canning CG. Recurrent Falls in Parkinson's Disease: A Systematic Review. Parkinson's Disease, Volume 2013, Article ID 906274, 16 pages.

906 http://www.cdc.gov/traumaticbraininjury/severe.html Accessed November 1, 2013.

907 Chapuis S, et al. Impact of the motor complications of Parkinson's disease on the quality of life. Movement Disorders, Volume 20, Issue 2, February 2005, Pages 224-230.

908 Gallagher DA, Lees AJ, Schrag A. What are the most important nonmotor symptoms in patients with Parkinson's disease and are we missing them? Movement Disorders, Volume 25, Issue 15, October 2010.

909 Cano de la Cuerda R, et al. Axial rigidity and quality of life in patients with Parkinson's disease: a preliminary study. Quality of Life Research volume 20, p. 817–823, 2011.

910 Kasten M, et al. Depression and quality of life in monogenic compared to idiopathic, early-onset Parkinson's disease. Movement Disorders, Volume 27, Issue 6, May 2012, Pages 754-759.

911 Kuopio AM, et al. The quality of life in Parkinson's disease. Movement Disorders, Volume 15, Issue 2, March 2000, Pages 216-223

912 Gallagher DA, Lees AJ, Schrag A. What are the most important nonmotor symptoms in patients with Parkinson's disease and are we missing them? Movement Disorders, Volume 25, Issue 15, October 2010.

913 Ongun N. Does nutritional status affect Parkinson's Disease features and quality of life? PLoS ONE 2018 13(10): e0205100

914 Van der Eijk M, et al. Moving from physician-centered care towards patient-centered care for Parkinson's disease patients. Parkinsonism and Related Disorders. http://dx.dxi.org/10.1016/j.parkreldis.2013.04.022

915 https://www.chcs.org/media/Health_Literacy_Implications_of_the_Affordable_Care_Act.pdf

Lightning Source UK Ltd.
Milton Keynes UK
UKHW021927121121
393874UK00008B/2158